CANCER ETIOLOGY, DIAGNOSIS AND TREATMENT

MAMMOGRAPHY

SCREENING, RESULTS AND RISKS

CANCER ETIOLOGY, DIAGNOSIS AND TREATMENT

Additional books in this series can be found on Nova's website under the Series tab.

Additional E-books in this series can be found on Nova's website under the E-book tab.

CANCER ETIOLOGY, DIAGNOSIS AND TREATMENT

MAMMOGRAPHY

SCREENING, RESULTS AND RISKS

ANDREA PALMETTI
AND
RAPHAËL ROUX
EDITORS

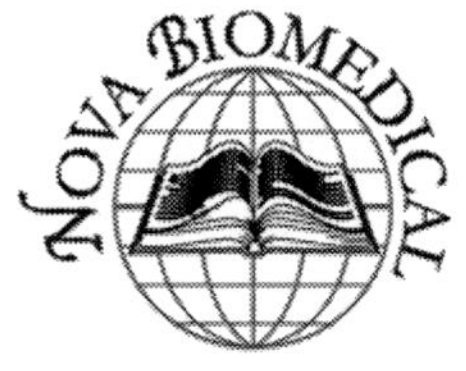

Nova Science Publishers, Inc.
New York

For permission to use material from this book please contact us:
Telephone 631-231-7269; Fax 631-231-8175
Web Site: http://www.novapublishers.com

Additional color graphics may be available in the e-book version of this book.

Library of Congress Cataloging-in-Publication Data

Mammography : screening, results, and risks / editors, Andrea Palmetti and Raphakl Roux.
p. ; cm.
Includes bibliographical references and index.
ISBN 978-1-61470-589-5 (hardcover : alk. paper) 1. Breast--Radiography. I. Palmetti, Andrea. II. Roux, Raphakl, 1967-
[DNLM: 1. Mammography. WP 815]
LC-classification not assigned
618.1'907572--dc23

2011025516

Published by Nova Science Publishers, Inc. † New York

CONTENTS

PREFACE

This book presents topical research in the study of mammography screening, results and risks. Topics discussed in this compilation include the socioeconomic and healthcare supply statistical determinants of compliance to mammography screening programs; digital breast tomosynthesis; the role of mammography in the reduction mammoplasty patient; mammography research in Thailand and a GIS approach to the access of mammography facilities and the detection of breast cancer.

Chapter 1- Although Asian American women have lower breast cancer incidence than white and black women (National Cancer Institute, National Institutes of Health [NIH], 2010) and lower mortality rates than any other U.S. racial/ethnic group (American Cancer Society, 2009), the rate of decline in invasive breast cancer incidence and mortality is lower than for any other group. From 1998 to 2007, for example, invasive breast cancer incidence in Asian/Pacific Islander (API) women decreased by only 0.4% compared to 1.7% for white women and 1.5% for all U.S. women. Similarly, from 2003 to 2007, breast cancer mortality declined by 1.9 per 100,000 persons for all U.S. women, but only 0.8% for API women less than any other group (Altekruse et al., 2010). In addition, research has indicated that cancer risks increase for Asian immigrant women with increased time in residence in the United States (Choi et al., 2010; Ma, Shive, Wang, & Tan, 2009). Suggested reasons for this increase include changes in lifestyle (e.g., later marriage, later pregnancy, diminished breastfeeding) as well as increased access to screening and diagnostic resources (Choi et al., 2010),

Chapter 2- X-ray mammography (both digital and film-screen) is considered the most effective imaging modality for detecting the early stages of breast cancer. However, it can not separately identify overlying tissue, which results in anatomical noise. This kind of noise is one of the biggest obstacles to the interpretation of mammograms and results in a considerable number of wrong diagnoses. Breast tomosynthesis emerged as a refinement of digital mammography, attempting to overcome this limitation by acquiring several projection images at different angular positions around a fixed point close to the centre of the detector. Series of 2D slice images of the breast are then reconstructed from these projections. However, the number of projections acquired is limited by the total dose which should be comparable to that used in conventional mammography. Commercial versions of tomosynthesis systems for breast imaging are now very close to market approval.

Chapter 3- Breast cancer is the main cause of mortality by cancer in women in France, responsible for 11,308 deaths in 2005, and the second cause of mortality by cancer in women in the United Kingdom, responsible for 11,990 deaths in 2007. Randomized controlled trials have demonstrated that mammography screening reduces breast cancer mortality by 21%. Similarly to many developed countries, except the United States, an organized breast cancer screening (BCS) program using mammography was set up in France in 1989, throughout 10 of the country's 96 geographical areas, referred to as ''departments''. This program was set up in 1996 in the Department of Calvados. In the French program, local screening management structures invited the target population, women aged from 50 to 74 years, by post to undergo a free mammography once every 2 years. Despite regular progress since the organized BCS program was generalized to include the entire French territory in 2004, the national rate of participation (52.5% in 2008) remains below European recommendations which advocate a 70% participation rate in order to obtain a significant reduction in mortality. Although the literature on factors associated with mammography screening is abundant, the reasons for underparticipation remain unclear, most studies having focused exclusively on individual factors. The use of screening mammography has been described in previous conceptual models as being influenced by both individual and environmental characteristics. Over the last decade, research has highlighted the influence of place of residence on behavior regarding screening, in particular BCS, and has increased awareness on the importance of considering ecological factors when studying individual behavior. Whereas individual-level socioeconomic influence has been firmly established, influence of socioeconomic status (SES) of place of residence is conflicting across studies. Certain studies have reported that women in areas with higher SES, such as higher median incomes, higher rate of being gainfully employed or higher school diplomas demonstrated higher utilization rates. On the contrary, in other studies, no employment–population ratio influence was observed. Findings regarding healthcare supply are also conflicting. Certain studies have reported that residing in a county with a greater number of physicians is associated with increased mammography, others observing no physician consultation rate influence. To study influence of socioeconomic status of place of residence on behavior regarding screening with predictor variables measured simultaneously at different levels, multilevel analysis is pertinent. Indeed, taking into account the hierarchical structure of data, multilevel analysis allows to obtain more exact estimations of area-level variance than classical analysis. A number of North American and Swedish studies on ecological SES influencing screening mammography participation have used multilevel analysis. Almost all of these studies were based on self-questionnaires on screening participation and were limited by participation bias; only the Swedish study was population-based. However, this last study on uptake within an organized screening program did not take into account healthcare supply in its multilevel analysis. The aim of this study was to investigate if area-level SES and area-level healthcare supply were independent predictors of non-adherence to an organized mammography screening program within a representative sample of the target population, after controlling for individual characteristics using multilevel models.

Chapter 4- There are many applications of classical X ray techniques in the present day. Some applications are developed in order to serve specific purpose. A technique called "mammography" is an application in this category. Mammography is a useful tool for searching of breast abnormality [1 – 5]. This is a kind of X ray study focusing on the breast, a specific organ of human body. The detection of abnormal calcification within breast tissue is an important principle concept of mammography. At present, this investigation plays important role in reduction of rate of breast malignancy in many countries. Although there are many reports on some limitations of the mammography, this tool is still accepted for its clinical usefulness. It is an actual hope to fight breast cancer.

Chapter 5- Of all plastic surgery procedures, reduction mammoplasty has one of the highest satisfaction rates. Over 200,000 women of all ages undergo this procedure each year in the United States. The Surveillance Epidemiology and End Results (SEER) database estimated that in 2009, 190,000 women would be diagnosed with breast cancer, and over 40,000 women would die of the disease . Screening mammography can detect asymptomatic early stage breast cancer, but despite the popularity of breast reduction surgery and the commonness of breast cancer, there is no standardized, accepted means of using mammography for evaluating reduction mammoplasty patients before surgery, or following these patients long-term for screening and diagnostic purposes. This lack of guidance has led to an assortment of different approaches by surgeons in their use of mammography in this patient

Chapter 6- Breast cancer is a major public health problem and the second leading cause of cancer death in the United States. In 2009, it is estimated that more than 254,000 women were diagnosed with breast cancer and more than 40,000 women died from this disease (American Cancer Society, 2009), including approximate 192,370 new invasive cases (i.e., late-stage cases) and 62,280 cases of in situ breast cancer (i.e., early stage cases). The use of mammography has been effective for detecting the early malignancies and has significantly reduced breast cancer mortality (Breen et al., 2007; Elkin et al., 2010). Previous studies indicated that each year 4,475 deaths from breast cancer could be prevented if all eligible Americans received cancer screening services (Baron et al., 2008; Institute of Medicine, 2003). The prevalence of mammography among women with ages equal to or older than 40 years, however, has declined in recent years and caused the concern for increased cancer mortality (Barton, 2001; Breen et al., 2007).

Chapter 7- Breast cancer is one of the leading causes of death among women in the United States. The American Cancer Society estimated that 178,480 new cases and 40,460 deaths from breast cancer occurred among women in the United States in 2007 (American Cancer Society [ACS], 2007). Due to a lack of primary prevention of breast cancer, breast cancer mortality and morbidity reduction depends on secondary prevention, chiefly through screening mammography. Several randomized trials as well as population-based screening evaluations have indicated that early detection of breast cancer through screening mammography improves treatment options, the likelihood of successful treatment, and improved survival (William, Holladay, and Sheikh 2003; Taber et al., 2003; Humphrey, Helfand, Chan, and Woolf, 2002; Duffy, Tabar, and Chen, 2002). A rise in mammography utilization is suggested by the observed trends (1987-1999) of an increase in breast cancer incidence confined to early stage breast cancer (Howe, et al., 2001; Edwards, et al., 2002; Blanchard, et al. 2004). A significant and substantial reduction in female breast cancer mortality has been observed in recent years because of screening mammography (Smith, et al., 2003; Duffy et al., 2006). However, the mortality rate from breast cancer is still too high, even though screening rates have increased and mortality decreased somewhat. The Healthy People 2010 target is 22.3 deaths per 100,000 women, but according to the American

Cancer Society data the death rate is 26 per 100,000 women in 2007 (ACS, 2007).

In: Mammography:
Editors: A. Palmetti, R. Roux

ISBN 978-1-61470-589-5

Chapter 1

FACTORS INFLUENCING MAMMOGRAPHY SCREENING PARTICIPATION AMONG THAI WOMEN IN SOUTHERN CALIFORNIA

Bulaporn Natipagon-Shah[1][1] ***and Mary Jo Clark***[2][2]

[1] School of Nursing, Azusa Pacific University
San Diego Regional Center, U. S.
5353 Mission Center Road Suite # 300
San Diego, CA, U. S.
[2] Hahn School of Nursing and Health Science
University of San Diego
5998 Alcala Park
San Diego, CA, U. S.

ABSTRACT

Purpose: To determine mammography participation and the prevalence of and interrelationships among factors influencing screening among Thai women living in southern California.

[1] E-mail address: bnatipagonshah@apu.edu
[2] E-mail address: clark@sandiego.edu

Background: Asian women as a group have lower rates of breast cancer incidence than other racial/ethnic groups, yet they typically experience lower survival rates due to later stage at diagnosis. Mammography screening rates are relatively low among this population (Centers for Disease Control and Prevention [CDC], 2010), and one study of Thai women in Los Angeles found that only 59% had received a mammogram in the prior two years (Thai Community Development Center, 2004). Little is known of factors that influence screening in this subpopulation of Asian women. Knowledge of factors that influence the use of mammography by this group can be used to develop culturally appropriate interventions that promote earlier diagnosis of breast cancer and better prognosis.

Design: A descriptive correlational design was used to explore mammography use and related factors among Thai women living in southern California.

Methods: Cluster sampling was used to identify women over 40 years of age in southern California who self-identified as Thai. Telephone interviews were conducted with 360 women using a questionnaire based on prior research regarding factors influencing mammography screening participation in this population.

Results: Several factors were reported as influencing mammography participation among Thai women living in southern California. Prior mammography use, frequency of use, and intent to obtain a mammogram in the next 12 months were associated with perceptions of breast cancer and associated risk, years in the United States, increasing age, health insurance, and having a regular health care provider.

Conclusions: Culturally appropriate interventions to promote breast cancer screening among Thai women in southern California should address identified influencing factors. For example, education should address misperceptions of low breast cancer risk, and interventions should particularly target younger women and recent immigrants.

INTRODUCTION

Although Asian American women have lower breast cancer incidence than white and black women (National Cancer Institute, National Institutes of Health [NIH], 2010) and lower mortality rates than any other U.S. racial/ethnic group (American Cancer Society, 2009), the rate of decline in invasive breast cancer incidence and mortality is lower than for any other group. From 1998 to

2007, for example, invasive breast cancer incidence in Asian/Pacific Islander (API) women decreased by only 0.4% compared to 1.7% for white women and 1.5% for all U.S. women. Similarly, from 2003 to 2007, breast cancer mortality declined by 1.9 per 100,000 persons for all U.S. women, but only 0.8% for API women less than any other group (Altekruse et al., 2010). In addition, research has indicated that cancer risks increase for Asian immigrant women with increased time in residence in the United States (Choi et al., 2010; Ma, Shive, Wang, & Tan, 2009). Suggested reasons for this increase include changes in lifestyle (e.g., later marriage, later pregnancy, diminished breastfeeding) as well as increased access to screening and diagnostic resources (Choi et al., 2010),

Late diagnosis and subsequent breast cancer mortality are often the result of failure to participate in breast cancer screening. Recent data indicate that Asian women in the United States are less likely than any other group to receive a mammogram in the prior two years. In 2008, for example, 65% of Asian women over 40 years of age had had a mammogram in the past two years compared to 76% of all U.S. women (National Centers for Chronic Disease Prevention and Health Promotion, 2009; Centers for Disease Control and Prevention [CDC], 2010). Asian immigrant women are even less likely to receive mammograms.

Asian-American Women and Mammography

U.S. breast cancer statistics are usually aggregated for the diverse ethnic groups that form the API population, in part because monolingual residents are often excluded from national surveys designed to identify health risks (Ma et al., 2009). This aggregation makes it difficult to identify factors that contribute to incidence or impede screening in specific Asian subpopulations. Culturally sensitive health promotion programs, however, require interventions that are adapted and tailored to the specific cultural mores and risk factors present in a given population. Recently, attempts have been made to disaggregate breast cancer information for selected subgroups. For example, an integrative review found studies of Chinese, Korean, Filipino, and Asian Indian women (Wu, Bancroft, & Guthrie, 2005). The authors concluded that, although demographic correlates of mammography screening had been identified, few studies addressed the cognitive and sociocultural influences on screening participation among these groups. Similarly, Sadler, Takahashi, Ko, and Nguyen (2003) examined breast cancer screening attitudes and behaviors among Japanese American women and found that participation in mammography increased with age. Barriers to screening identified by study participants included lack of time, cost, and unwillingness to think about breast cancer or lack of perceived importance of screening. Sadler et al. also noted that effective breast cancer intervention programs must be tailored to the beliefs, values, and circumstances of Asian ethnic groups.

Studies of other groups of Asian American women indicate a variety of factors that impede breast cancer screening. For example, Yu and associates (2002) identified cultural, psychosocial, linguistic, and economic barriers to breast and cervical cancer screening among Asian women. Gilani and Kamal (2004) studied biological risk factors (BMI, family history, parity, consanguinity, age at menarche, age at first pregnancy, and history of abortion) and their association with breast cancer incidence in Pakistani women, but did not address possible factors influencing screening participation. Facione, Giancarlo, & Chan (2000) examined cultural beliefs and behaviors as they related to breast cancer screening intentions among Chinese-American women and found a number of factors that influenced screening and diagnostic behaviors. An older study among Vietnamese and Cambodian women in Philadelphia (Phipps, Cohen, Sorn, & Braitman, 1999) found little knowledge of cancer or preventive measures for breast and cervical cancer in this population, and Sadler et al. (2001) reported that Asian Indian women indicated low levels of knowledge about breast cancer as an impediment to screening.

More recent studies have continued to explore the salience of various factors in mammography participation decisions among different groups of Asian women in the United States. For example, Wu and Bancroft (2006) found that screening behaviors among Filipino women were influenced by support from family members, health insurance reinforcement and virtual mandate, recommendations from familiar physicians (particularly women physicians who spoke the clients' language), presence of abnormal breast symptoms, a family history or personal diagnosis of breast cancer, and health literacy in the form of knowledge about breast cancer and the need for screening. Barriers to screening were identified as differing uses of mammography for diagnostic purposes in the Philippines and use as a screening tool in the United States, cost and accessibility, lack of knowledge of insurance coverage of services, and inaccurate knowledge of screening measures. More personal barriers included pain and discomfort related to past mammography experiences, reluctance to think about cancer, and fear that having the test would lead to occurrence of the disease. Filipino women also expressed cultural reluctance to exposing their breasts and having them touched and logistical barriers to screening such as difficulties with scheduling, transportation, and lack of knowledge of local screening resources.

Like Wu and Bancroft, Ma and associates (2009), found that having a physician who spoke one's native language was associated with higher rates of screening participation. They suggested that this might occur because physicians who do not speak the client's primary language may have limited skills in the language or rely on untrained interpreters increasing the potential for misunderstanding of messages about screening. Having a physician of the same ethnicity, however, was found to be correlated with not receiving mammography services among Asian Indian women in the United States (Somanchi, Juon, & Rimal, 2010). Not having a regular health care provider, was also associated with lack of participation in mammography in this population. Additional barriers to screening participation reported by the women included not having any breast problems, cost and lack of insurance, laziness, beliefs that mammography was not needed, and lack of time. Interestingly, more than a fourth of the women (28.9%) indicated that there was no particular reason they had not had a mammogram. Factors that contributed to screening participation, on the other hand, included being married, more years in the United States, being knowledgeable about screening guidelines, being between 50 and 64 years of age, health insurance coverage, and participation of relatives in mammography screening.

Su, Ma, Seals, Tan, and Hausman (2006) conducted a study of breast cancer screening behavior among Chinese women in Philadelphia and found that the only significant predictor of mammography participation in multivariate analysis was having a physician as a source of information on screening. Women in the study, however, indicated that knowledge about mammography and of local services, free services, and availability of Chinese interpreters, as well as physician recommendation, were motivating factors in screening. Barriers to screening identified by this group included feeling well/not having any breast symptoms, lack of facility with English, and cost.

Two recent studies were found examining breast cancer screening participation among Korean American women. In a study by Lee, Kim, and Han (2009), cultural factors, such as modesty and use of Eastern medicine, were correlated with mammography participation among Korean American women with good English skills, while only modesty was related to participation among those with limited facility with English. Perceived benefits of mammography and perceived susceptibility to breast cancer were also related to screening participation. In another study, only age was found to be a significant predictor of mammography screening participation, with Korean American women aged 50 to 64 years being more likely than younger women to have had a mammogram in the past 2 years. Education was also marginally significant, with higher educational levels related to greater participation Although not significant in multivariate analyses, education, English proficiency, health insurance, and self-reports of good to excellent health were significantly associated with mammography participation in bivariate analyses. Several other variables were linked with screening participation among Korean women in Korea, suggesting a change in influencing factors after immigration (Choi et al., 2010).

Wu and Ronis (2009) explored correlates of mammography screening among Asian-American women born in China/Taiwan, Korea. India, and the Philippines, but did not differentiate findings by ethnic group. Among the sample at large, however, they found that knowledge of screening recommendations, length of time in the United States, and facility with English were associated with regular mammography participation, while women with more reported barriers to screening were less likely to participate in regular screening as recommended. The authors did not, however, indicate the frequency of responses for particular barriers included in the perceived barriers scale.

Glenn, Chawla, Surani, & Bastani (2009) examined factors involved in participation in several cancer screening modalities among South Asians, immigrants from India, Pakistan, Sri Lanka, Bangladesh, Nepal, Bhutan, and the Maldives. Due to small sample sizes for other populations, multivariate analyses of factors influencing screening were conducted only on data from Indian, Pakistani, Bangladeshi, and Sri Lankan participants and reported only in the aggregate except for mammography screening frequency which was most common among Indians. Factors found to be associated with mammography participation included insurance status, age, and years in the United States. Unlike Choi et al. (2010) and Somanchi et al. (2010), they found younger people more likely to have received mammograms than older ones, a finding consistent with the general U. S. population (CDC, 2010).

Studies have also been done exploring acculturation and mammography screening among Hispanic women (Fernandez, Palmer, & Leong-Wu, 2005; Palmer, Fernandez, Tortolero-Luna, Gonzales, & Mullen, 2005) and strategies to promote screening in African American women (Fernandez, et al., 2005; Garza et al., 2005) and native Hawaiian women (Ka`opua & Anngela, 2005). Few studies, however, have been conducted among Thai women in the United States, and incidence and prevalence figures for this population are not available. Nor is there information on the extent of participation of Thai women in mammography screening programs or on the factors that promote or impede their participation.

Breast Cancer and Thai Women

Given the lack of information on cancer incidence and prevalence and mammography screening among Thai women in the United States, incidence and prevalence figures for Thailand may serve to suggest the magnitude of disease among this population in the United States. Although breast cancer incidence in Thailand is lower than in many other countries , it is the most common form of cancer among Thai women (International Agency for Research on Cancer, 2008). This is a change from 1996, when cervical cancer incidence was higher than breast cancer incidence (19.5 vs. 17.2 cases per 100,000 women) (Martin & Patel, 2003). In 2008, the incidence rate for breast cancer among women in Thailand was 30.7 per 100,000 women, and the mortality rate was 10.8, less only than the mortality rate for liver cancer (16.6 per 100,000) and cervical cancer (12.8 per 100,000) (International Agency for Research on Cancer, 2008), In addition, breast cancer incidence has been increasing in Thailand. For example, from 1990 to 1999, incidence increased from 13.5 per 100,000 women to 19.8 (Ministry of Public Health [MOPH], n.d.a).

Breast cancer in Thailand also occurs at younger ages than in the United States, with a peak age at diagnosis of 35 years in Thailand, suggesting a particular need to promote mammography screening in younger women in this population (Wilailak, 2009). From 2005 to 2007, 55% of breast cancer diagnoses in Thailand occurred in women under 50 years of age, while 77% of diagnoses occurred in this age group in the United States (MOPH, n.d.b). Incidence at younger ages among Thai women was also supported by a case-control study conducted by Jordan and associates (2009).

In addition, breast cancer diagnosis tends to occur at more advanced stages among Thai women than among U.S. women. From 2000 to 2007 among U.S. women, for example, 61% of breast cancer diagnoses are made at the localized stage (National Cancer Institute, Institutes of Health, n.d.). In Thailand, on the other hand, 80% of breast cancer diagnoses from 2005 to 2007 were invasive cancers (MOPH, n.d.b). Although breast cancer incidence in Thailand and among Thai women in the United States may differ significantly, the recent increase in breast cancer diagnoses in Thailand suggests the need to obtain information on breast cancer and screening participation among this population in the United States.

U.S. Thai Women and Mammography Screening

The actual number of Thai women in the United States is unknown due to the number of undocumented persons who have entered the U.S. legally and then overstayed their visa limits. The 2000 census documented 169,800 persons in the United States born in Thailand, 68% of whom were women over 20 years of age (U. S. Census Bureau, 2000). In 2007, the Thai consulate in Los Angeles reported approximately 130,000 Thai in Los Angeles County alone. Again, approximately two thirds of this population is women. A report by the Thai Community Development Center (2004), indicated that only 59% of Thai women over 40 years of age in the Los Angeles area had received a mammogram in the previous two years, less than the percentage of U.S. Asian women or women in the general population.

Little is known about the reasons for low levels of breast cancer screening in the Thai population. Studies in Thailand have indicated that the availability and geographic distribution of mammography services may influence screening participation, particularly in rural areas (Putthasri, Tangcharoensathien, Mugem, & Jindawatana, 2004). In addition, a number of social and health system variables have been shown to influence delay in receiving care for breast cancer (Thongsuksai, Chongsuvivatwong, & Sriplung, 2000) and may also influence screening participation. Whether similar factors are operating in the U. S. Thai population is unknown. Kumsuk (2005) conducted a series of three focus groups with Thai women in the Midwestern United States and found perceptions of breast cancer and mammography screening similar to those of non-Asian groups, but also found distinctly Thai perceptions that influenced screening participation. These included the belief that mammography flattens the breast, that "healthy women" do not need mammograms, and that the likelihood of developing breast cancer is predetermined and cannot be changed. Participants indicated a need for culturally appropriate materials written in Thai to educate this population about the need for mammograms. In a later study, Kumsuk (2006) used tools based on the Health Belief Model, an acculturation scale, and an Asian value scale to create a Thai Breast Cancer Belief Scale. The tool was used to identify stages of change related to mammography participation among Thai women in the Midwest. The rate of mammography participation noted in

Kumsuk's 2006 study was even lower than that for Asian American women in general. Placement in the action/maintenance stage of change was associated with an awareness of the seriousness of breast cancer, adoption of an Americanized lifestyle, and self-identification as American rather than Thai.

Due to the paucity of information on mammography participation among Thai women in southern California, the authors of this chapter undertook a preliminary phenomenological study to describe breast cancer screening participation from the perspective of those experiencing the phenomenon (Clark & Natipagon-Shah, 2008). Phenomenology deals with participants' lived experience of the phenomena of interest (Groenewald, 2004).

The study employed a series of focus groups with women in the Thai communities in Los Angeles and San Diego Counties to identify factors that influenced screening. Focus groups were used because of their potential for identifying beliefs, values, and perceptions prevalent in a population. The study was approved by an Institutional Review Board, and written informed consent was obtained prior to each focus group. Participants were given a $25 gift card in appreciation of their participation.

Women 40 years of age or older, who self-identified as Thai, living in Los Angeles and San Diego counties were included in the study. Participants included both Thai and English-speaking women with or without a history of breast cancer. Women were recruited from two community services agencies serving the Thai populations in Los Angeles and San Diego counties. Congruent with a phenomenological approach, purposive sampling was used to identify women likely be knowledgeable, by virtue of their positions in the community, about screening behaviors in the population. Participants identified by agency personnel as being knowledgeable about the Thai community and Thai culture were personally invited to participate by the Thai member of the research team. A total of 70 women were invited to participate to assure adequate sampling and account for last minute inability to participate. Forty women agreed to participate in the study. Women who chose not to participate reported lack of time as their reasons for doing so, rather than a reluctance to discuss the topic.

Initially, the group targeted for participation in the focus groups was women over 50 years of age because of the trend for decreased mammography participation with increasing age in the general U. S. population. Data from early focus groups, however, indicated that the opposite trend was present in the Thai population in southern California, with older women more likely to obtain mammograms than younger women. For that reason, participants between 40 and 50 years of age were purposefully recruited for later focus groups.

Four focus groups lasting one and a half to two hours and comprised of 6 to 11 participants were conducted The focus groups were conducted in Thai, English, and a combination of both, based on participants' choice. Both investigators participated in focus group facilitation, with the native Thai-speaking investigator serving as translator during portions of focus groups conducted in Thai. Her facility with both Thai and English permitted group participants to convey their thoughts in ways in which they were most comfortable, but also allowed the more experienced researcher, who did not speak Thai, to assist in directing probes and asking for expansion and clarification of ideas presented.

Focus group participants were asked about their own screening participation and why they had decided to have or not have a mammogram. They were asked similar questions about factors influencing screening participation by family members and friends. Follow-up probes were used to elicit additional information as needed. Analysis of early transcripts led to additional questions to validate and clarify preliminary concepts. Field notes were recorded during each focus group session describing the participants, interaction, and major concepts addressed, and theoretical memos were written after each session.

Thirty-six women participated in the focus groups. Most participants (89%) were over 50 years of age, with an age range of 40 to 73 years. Participants had been in the United States from a few years to decades, but all were born outside of the U.S. Two thirds of the women were retired; others worked in local Thai restaurants and other businesses, in nursing or teaching, or were self-employed.

Participants were actively involved in the focus groups with considerable give and take of ideas. Data analysis was ongoing and involved thematic analysis of transcriptions of the audio-taped focus group sessions. The Thai-speaking investigator translated the transcriptions from Thai to English as needed. Accuracy of translations was corroborated with independent translations by a native Thai-speaking doctoral student in nursing. Data saturation was achieved after four focus groups and no further themes or concepts were identified.

Data analysis included the identification of themes and categories of factors believed by participants to influence mammography screening participation, either positively or negatively. Data analysis was conducted separately by each of the investigators and the findings compared and discussed until agreement was reached. Following initial analysis, the findings were presented for validation to members of the Thai community, several of whom who had participated in the focus groups. Community members agreed that findings accurately represented factors influencing screening participation.

Overall categories of factors influencing mammography screening included perceptions of cancer, encouragement, health consciousness, physical factors, fear, cultural factors, social responsibilities, and logistical barriers. Findings related to each category are addressed briefly below.

Perceptions

Accurate knowledge and misinformation about breast cancer and breast cancer screening had contrasting effects on screening participation. Participants indicated that lack of knowledge about breast cancer and the importance of mammography for early diagnosis impeded mammography participation. Awareness of family members with a diagnosis of breast cancer was a motivator for participation. Conversely, several women who did not know of any family history of breast cancer felt they did not need regular mammograms.

Misperceptions about breast cancer incidence and prevalence among Thai women were other reasons for not receiving a mammogram. Women repeatedly voiced the perception that “Thai people don’t get cancer much” and that it was “not in our nature.” Interestingly, the majority of the women knew at least one Thai woman who had been diagnosed with breast cancer yet still perceived decreased susceptibility compared to other American women.

Other misinformation was reported as influencing Thai women’s participation in mammography. For example, many women voiced the perception that only older women got cancer. Another misperception voiced by women in the study was that women who are healthy do not need mammograms. A few other women believed that a normal mammogram in the past meant they did not need subsequent screening unless they developed symptoms.

Further misperceptions centered on the contribution of marriage and sexual intercourse to one’s risk of breast cancer. Some women felt that fondling the breasts during intercourse increased one’s risk of cancer and that prostitutes might be at greater risk because they “get squeezed a lot.” A few women believed that mammography itself might actually cause cancer because of the compression of the breasts during the procedure. Most, however, believed that although mammography is uncomfortable, it does not cause cancer.

One area of misinformation reported has resulted from a consistent health provider focus on teaching breast self-examination (BSE) to their clients. Many of the women still perceived BSE as an effective method of detecting breast cancer despite the findings of the U.S. Preventive Services Task Force (2009b) to the contrary. Some women who did not obtain mammograms reported that they did not need to because they engaged in regular BSE and perceived it to be an effective substitute for detecting disease.

Finally, knowledge of the availability of mammography services and how to access them was believed to facilitate participation. Conversely, not knowing where to obtain mammography services was seen as an impediment to screening.

Encouragement

The women participating in the focus groups described encouragement as a major factor in decisions to obtain a mammogram. Recommendations of both health care providers and friends or family members were described as motivating mammography participation, and some women suggested that without a recommendation from their providers they would probably not have obtained a mammogram. Several women reported encouraging other Thai women to be screened.

A few women suggested that providers' recommendations that they not get a mammogram were a deciding factor. In some cases, this recommendation was based on the woman's age, but one woman was told she did not need a mammogram because she had had a hysterectomy. Another woman reported misinformation provided by a nurse family member that mammography was not necessary and might cause breast trauma and subsequent cancer.

Health Consciousness

Being conscious of one's health was another reason given for obtaining a mammogram. Health consciousness tended to be mentioned as a result of menopause. Changes in bodily function and appearance were seen as potential signs of other possible changes such as breast cancer. Some perimenopausal and postmenopausal women described their response as wanting to "keep what we have" in the face of other changes.

Physical Factors

A variety of physical factors were also reported as influencing mammography participation. For example, large breast size was seen as a contributing factor in breast cancer development, but women with smaller breasts saw themselves as at less risk for disease. Similarly, breast augmentation was viewed as an indication of the need for mammography. Other changes in the breast, such as lumps, pain, or fluid leaking from the nipples, were also suggested as reasons why Thai women would obtain a mammogram.

Pain was also reported as a deterrent to mammography, and several women cited the attendant discomfort as a reason for not participating in screening. Others described the pain associated with mammography as a reason for putting it off, although they reported that they eventually got screened.

Fear

Fear was reported as both a facilitator for and an impediment to breast cancer screening. Women who perceived themselves as at risk for breast cancer and feared developing it wished to find out as early as possible to support a good treatment outcome. Many women, however, described a general fear of cancer and not wanting to know if they had it as reasons why Thai women did not get mammograms. Others also suggested that just thinking about the disease and having the tests might lead to developing cancer.

Cultural Factors

The most common cultural factor influencing mammography participation was a cultural reticence to expose one's breasts. The women in the focus groups reported that one's breasts were not a topic for conversation and that even same sex siblings had never seen each other's breasts. They also indicated that they were not encouraged to think about their own breasts. Several of the women suggested that this “cultural shyness” diminished with age and with length of residence in the United States.

Belief in karma was the second cultural barrier to mammography screening reported by the women in the study. They noted that many Thai women may see developing breast cancer as their fate and believe that screening is futile. Such “cancer fatalism” has been noted in other ethnic cultural groups and is not unique to Thai women (Brooks, Hamilton, & Powe, 2006; Burgess, Linsell, & Ramirez, 2008; Powe, 1995).

Social Responsibilities

Another category of barriers to mammography participation involved competing social responsibilities. Women were reported as having multiple family and work responsibilities that left them with no time for screening services. Work responsibilities were compounded by the fact that most of them worked in low-paying service jobs with schedules inconsistent with mammography screening services. They also noted that many Thai women could not afford to ask for time off to participate in screening and suggested that employers be mandated to permit use of work time for screening activities such as mammography. Some older women indicated that their retirement and no longer being responsible for raising families left them more time to focus on their own health needs, including breast cancer screening.

Logistical Barriers

Logistical barriers to breast cancer screening reported by women in the focus groups included cost, lack of health insurance, and language barriers. Many women could not afford the cost of mammography services and worked in jobs that did not include health insurance benefits. Even when they were aware of free or low-cost mammography services available in some areas, scheduling of services was difficult given the work and family responsibilities described above.

Some women who were not fluent in English described language barriers as a deterrent to screening. They noted that interpreters were often not available and they needed to bring family members to translate for them. This often necessitated the family member, as well as the client, asking for time off work. A few women also mentioned the problem of not adequately understanding the prescreening instructions for having a mammogram and having to return because they had used deodorant prior to being screened. In addition, a few women described distance to screening services as a logistical barrier.

THE CURRENT STUDY

The focus group study described above (Clark & Natipagon-Shah, 2008) provided some insight into factors that may contribute to low mammography screening rates among Thai women in the United States. We still did not, however, have any information on how prevalent these factors were among the Thai population in southern California. For that reason, we designed a follow-up study using telephone surveys to determine the prevalence of these factors and their relationships to mammography screening in this population.

Study Purpose and Research Questions

The purpose of the current study was to determine the extent to which factors influencing breast cancer screening identified in the focus groups were present among Thai women in southern California. Specific study questions included the following:

1. What is the extent of mammography participation among Thai women living in southern California?
2. To what extent are factors identified as motivating or impeding mammography participation present in the population?
3. What are the relationships between these factors and mammography participation?

Conceptual Framework

Because of its fit with the findings of the prior focus group study, the Health Belief Model (HBM) was used as the conceptual framework for the current study. The HBM was developed by Hochbaum, Kegeles, Leventhal, & Rosenstock (Green, 1974), and has been consistently used to study health behavior motivation since then. The origins of HBM lie in Lewin's field theory of change, in which positive and negative forces promote or impede, respectively, an individual's decision to engage in a particular behavior.

The HBM framed these forces in terms of beliefs held by the individual about the behavior and its consequences. Later testing of the model indicated that even in the presence of beliefs that promoted healthful behavior, some people did not act without a definite cue to action. Other variables or modifying factors were also found to influence one's ability to take action (e.g., age, education, income). In the model, beliefs that influence health-related behavior include beliefs about one's susceptibility to the problem addressed by the behavior, the perceived seriousness of the problem, and perceptions regarding the benefits of and barriers to engaging in the specific behavior - mammography screening in the case of this study (Rosenstock, 1974). Self-efficacy, or the perception that one is capable of performing the behavior is another component added to later versions of the model (Daddario, 2007).

The HBM has been used in studies related to a variety of personal health behaviors with ethnically diverse populations. For example, Daddario (2007) examined the use of the model in weight management programs, and Gatewood et al. (2008) found that perceived barriers and susceptibility and modifying factors such as transportation costs and work schedules influenced participation in a community-based cardiovascular risk reduction program. The HBM has also been used as a framework for studies of cancer screening participation. Guilfoyle, Franco, and Gorin (2007), for instance, found that perceived barriers and cues to action affected older women's participation in cervical cancer screening. The model has also been used in studies of mammography screening practices among older U.S. women (Menon et al., 2007), Chinese American immigrants (Lee-Lin et al., 2007), rural Turkish women (Avci & Kurt, 2008), and Korean women (Ham, 2007).

The HBM is particularly appropriate to the current study because factors identified by the focus group participants as influencing mammography screening among Thai women in southern California reflect several components of the model. For example, inaccurate beliefs about susceptibility include perceptions that Thai women are not at risk for breast cancer and that younger women and those who are healthy do not get breast cancer. Beliefs about the lack of benefits to screening were reflected in concepts of karma reported by the focus group participants, in which some women believed if they were fated to get cancer, it would not matter whether it was detected early or not. Other women who received mammograms, however, perceived benefit to early diagnosis and treatment.

A number of other barriers to screening also surfaced in the focus group interviews. For example, family and work responsibilities interfered with women's abilities to obtain mammograms. Other barriers included the pain of mammography itself, reticence to expose one's breasts, cost of and distance to services, and language difficulties and the resulting discomfort in health care situations. Being a more recent immigrant to the United States and knowledge about breast cancer and mammography availability were modifying factors that influenced screening participation. Finally, some women reported cues to action, such as a diagnosis of breast cancer in a friend or family member or physical changes in their breasts as motivating screening participation (Clark & Natipagon-Shah, 2008).

Methods

Design and sample. The study employed a descriptive correlational design using a telephone survey to address the research questions posed. Study participants included 360 women over 40 years of age living in southern California who self-identified as Thai. Because of the age of participants, all of the women were immigrants to the United States. Only younger women in this population tend to be native born.

Participants were initially recruited from lists of Thai women involved in activities at a major Thai social services center in the Los Angeles area and a Thai Buddhist temple in the San Diego area. Thereafter, a snowball sampling technique was used in which participants identified other women meeting the criteria who might be willing to participate in the study. Women invited to participate were informed of the purpose of the study, its voluntary nature, and that participation would not affect their receipt of services at any of the agencies involved in the study. An informed consent form was read to potential participants over the telephone and verbal consent to participate was obtained after any questions were answered. All participants were mailed a $10 gift card for a local department store in appreciation of their participation. Women who provided additional names and contact information were asked for permission to use their names when contacting subsequent participants.

Measurement. Data were collected in telephone interviews using an investigator-designed survey instrument. This tool was based on the findings of the prior focus group study that identified possible factors influencing mammography screening in the Thai immigrant population (Clark & Natipagon-Shah, 2008). The questionnaire consisted of five sections, the first of which asked for demographic data related to age, years of residence in the United States, health insurance status, and use of a regular health care provider and his or her ethnicity. This section also asked whether interviewees knew of family members or other Thai women with a diagnosis of breast cancer and solicited information on prior mammography experience and intentions to obtain a mammography in the next 12 months (rated from 1 to 4 as "no", "maybe no," "maybe yes", and "yes").

The second section of the questionnaire addressed participants' perceptions of and beliefs about breast cancer and the need for mammography. Items in this section were based on several areas of misperception identified in the focus groups. Items were scored from 4 for strong agreement with an accurate statement about breast cancer (e.g., "Mothers should tell their daughters to get a mammogram when they approach age 40," "Finding out about breast cancer early makes it easier to cure") to 1 for strong disagreement. Scoring was reversed for agreement or disagreement with inaccurate statements (e.g., "Thai women rarely get breast cancer," "Women who are healthy do not need a mammogram"). The range of agreement possible in the scoring system, as opposed to a yes/no response, was intended to elicit the degree of participants' certainty regarding a particular statement. The scores on the 14 items were then summed to create an overall score that reflected more or less accurate perceptions about breast cancer. Higher overall scores indicated more accurate perceptions regarding breast cancer and breast cancer screening.

The third section of the instrument asked women to rate their agreement or disagreement with statements about factors that might motivate mammography screening and circumstances when a woman should get a mammogram. A rating of 4 indicated that the participant strongly agreed with the statement as a reason for getting a mammogram, while a rating of 1 indicated strong disagreement that the factor was influential in motivating screening participation. Examples of items related to influencing factors include "The doctor recommends it," and "They are getting older and more conscious of their health." Examples of circumstances that might lead to mammography included "When they find a lump in their breasts" and "When they have big breasts." Again, the items were based on data derived from the focus group study.

Factors that might impede screening participation were addressed in the fourth section of the instrument. Questions addressed barriers identified by focus group participants such as the discomfort of the procedure, fear of finding out they have cancer, lack of time due to other responsibilities, shyness, lack of health insurance, and so on. Again, the interviewees were asked to rate their extent of agreement with each item as a barrier to mammography participation with 4 indicating strong agreement that the factor was influential and 1 indicating strong disagreement.

The fifth set of questions dealt with perceived causes of breast cancer such as trauma to the breast (accidental or caused by mammography), use of hormone replacement therapy (HRT), being sexually active, karma, and so on. Women were again asked to rate their level of agreement or disagreement with statements provided. Because items in sections 3, 4, and 5 were independent of each other, cumulative scores were not calculated for these sections. A final question asked about the respondent's intention of getting a mammogram in the next year. Responses were rated as 4 – "yes,", 3 – "maybe yes", 2 – "Maybe no," or 1 – "No."

The investigators followed universal guidelines for translating program materials and instruments developed by Eremenco, Cella, and Arnold (2005) in translating the survey tool into Thai. Recommended steps in the process include (a) translation into the target language by bilingual translators; (b) backward translation to compare the new document with the original; (c) review by the developer of the original document to ensure consistency; (d) pilot testing the translated document with members of the target population; and finally, (e) a second review by independent bilingual translators.

The instrument used in this study was developed by the authors based on the findings of the focus group interviews. It was then translated into Thai by the Thai-speaking investigator. The translation was back translated by another native Thai-speaking nurse and the resulting translation and suggested revisions were reviewed with the investigators. Then the Thai version was reviewed for clarity and cultural sensitivity by a group of community members who participated in the initial focus group study. Some changes in wording and scoring rubrics were made on the basis of their input. The revised instrument was pilot tested in telephone interviews with 15 women from the Thai community in Los Angeles and found to be understandable and culturally acceptable.

The final survey was used in telephone interviews with Thai women living in southern California. Interviews were conducted by three native Thai-speaking registered nurses. Attempts were made to contact a total of 487 women; of these, 44 or 9% were unable to be reached after three to five attempts. The remaining 443 women were successfully contacted, and 360 (81%) agreed to participate in the study. A total of 83 women declined to participate. Data on age and years in the United States were obtained for these women to determine their similarity or difference from participants. The two groups were similar on both variables. The mean age for non-participants was 53 years compared to 55 years for participants. With respect to U.S. residence, 29% of non-participants had been in the United States fewer than 10 years compared to 26% of participants. Surveys were conducted in either English or Thai as desired by the participants.

Data Analysis. Frequencies and percentages were used to examine sample characteristics, screening participation, and perceptions of breast cancer and breast cancer screening. T-tests assuming non-equal variance were used to explore differences between groups on specific factors (e.g., the difference in overall accuracy of perceptions regarding breast cancer and breast cancer screening between women who had and had not had a prior mammogram or between those with a Thai or non-Thai health care provider). The Mann-Whitney *U* was used to explore differences between women who had and had not had a prior mammogram and specific beliefs and perceptions about breast cancer and breast cancer screenings. Mann-Whitney *U* was also used to determine differences in frequency of mammography participation by age group and by years residing in the United States. Chi square was used to examine the relationships between having health insurance and mammography participation, having a regular health care provider and having had a mammogram, and having a regular health care provider and mammography frequency.

Spearman's rho correlations were used to examine associations between influencing factors and two of the three outcome variables of interest, frequency of mammography and intent to obtain a mammogram in the next 12 months). Spearman's rho provides correlations between data arranged in rank order. For purposes of statistical testing, for example, responses on the item related to mammography frequency were ranked 1 – "every year," 2 – "every 2-3 years," and 3 – "less often than every three years." Similarly, data related to years in the United States was categorized and ranked as 1 – "less than 5 years," 2 – "5 to 10 years," and 3 – "more than 10 years."

Findings

Study findings will be addressed in terms of participant characteristics, extent of mammography screening participation and intent to be screened, overall beliefs and perceptions about breast cancer and breast cancer screening, perceptions of factors promoting screening participation, and perceived barriers to screening. Then specific relationships among factors will be presented.

Characteristics of participants. A total of 360 women 40 to 81 years of age participated in the study. Characteristics of the sample are summarized in Table 1. The majority of the women (78%) were under 60 years of age, and 35% were under age 50. Nearly three fourths of the women (74%) had lived in the United States for more than 10 years, while 14 % had been here less than 5 years. As noted earlier, study participants did not differ from non-participants in either respect.

About half of the sample (56%) was insured by either public or private health insurance. Only 61% of the 297 women who responded to the item had a regular health care provider. Ninety-four percent of the women who had a regular health care provider responded regarding their providers' ethnicity, and 87% of these women saw providers who were not Thai.

Screening participation and intent. The women were asked about past mammography participation, frequency of mammography, and their intentions to obtain a mammogram in the next 12 months. Most of the women (84%) reported having had a mammogram at some time in their lives, but 16% had never had a mammogram. Slightly over half (56%) of those who had ever had the procedure and who reported on mammography frequency reported annual mammograms; 28% received a mammogram every 2 to 3 years; and 16% had obtained mammograms less often than every 3 years. Ninety-four percent of the women who responded to the item reported that they would or might get a mammogram in the next year. Mammography participation information is summarized in Table 2.

Beliefs and perceptions about breast cancer. The majority of the women had relatively high scores for the accuracy of their beliefs and perceptions about breast cancer and breast cancer screening in section 2 of the survey instrument. The mean score for this section of the instrument was 81%. A higher score for accuracy of perceptions about breast cancer and mammography was significantly correlated with age, with younger women exhibiting higher scores (r_s = 0.161, p. 0.01). Higher scores were also correlated with screening intentions in the coming year (r_s = 0.327, p. 0.01), but not with mammography frequency.

Table 1. Participant Characteristics

Characteristic	Number	Percent*
Age (N = 360)		
40-50 years	125	35%
51-60 years	154	43%
61-70 years	62	17%
> 70 years	19	5%
Years in U.S. (N = 360)		
< 5 years	50	14%
5-10 years	43	12%
> 10 years	257	74%
Health insurance (N = 356)		
Yes	198	56%
No	158	44%
Regular health care provider (N = 297)		
Yes	181	61%
No	116	39%
Provider ethnicity (N = 170)		
Thai	13	8%
Non-Thai	157	92%
Know Thai women with breast cancer diagnosis (N = 258)	208	58%
Yes	150	42%
No		
Family member with breast cancer (N = 359)		
Yes	35	10%
No	324	90%

*Due to rounding percents may not add to 100%

Items on which 20% or more of the women reported inaccurate perceptions dealt with Thai women's risk of developing breast cancer, breast cancer screening for older women, availability of free mammography services, the need for repeat mammography after a negative result, and the relationships among breast cancer development, marital status, and sexual intercourse. More than a third of the women (38%) agreed or strongly agreed with the statement that Thai women rarely get breast cancer, suggesting that perceptions of low risk may influence screening participation. This finding is particularly interesting in view of the fact that 58% of the respondents indicated that they knew at least one Thai woman who had been diagnosed with breast cancer.

Table 2. Prior Mammography Participation, Frequency, and Intention to Obtain a Mammogram

	Number	Percent*
Prior mammography participation (N = 360)		
Ever had a mammogram	304	84%**
Never had a mammogram	56	16%
Mammogram in the prior year	211	59%
Mammography frequency (N=298)		
Annual	166	56%
Every 2-3 years	84	28%
Less often than every 3 years	48	16%
Intention to obtain a mammogram (N = 358)		
Yes	239	66%
Maybe yes	92	26%
Maybe no	15	4%
No	12	3%

*Due to rounding percents may not add to 100%

** Includes those who reported a mammogram in the prior year

Similarly, 36% of the women believed that women over 70 years of age do not need mammograms. This finding is perhaps explained by news coverage of the controversy regarding guidelines for the age when routine mammography screening should be discontinued. Only three of four women were aware of free mammography screening services in the local area, suggesting a need to better publicize available services. Nearly one fifth of the respondents believed that if they had had a normal mammogram in the past, subsequent annual mammograms were not needed.

Approximately one in five women (21%) who answered believed that married women were at greater risk for breast cancer than single women. This was somewhat higher than the percentage of women who indicated that being married actually caused breast cancer in section 5 of the survey tool (5%). In section 2, 22% of the women agreed that not being sexually active decreased one's risk of breast cancer, while 8% of the women agreed that having sex caused breast cancer in section 5 of the tool. Specific aspects of sexual activity reported as causing cancer may explain the differences in the responses on these two items. Additional items in section 5 asked about squeezing or touch the breasts and prostitution as possible causes of cancer. Twenty-eight percent of the respondents agreed that "squeezing or touching the breasts too much" might cause cancer, and 29% agreed that prostitution was a cause of breast cancer. In the focus groups, women frequently equated excessive fondling or squeezing of the breasts with prostitution.

Other areas where some women expressed misperceptions were related to the relationship of breast size to breast cancer development, the need to get a mammogram even without a positive family history of disease, and beliefs about mammography as a cause of breast cancer and the protective effects of breastfeeding. Similar percentages of women agreed or strongly agreed that having small breasts decreased one's risk of breast cancer (13%) and that having a mammogram might itself cause breast cancer (15%). Conversely, in section 3 of the survey tool, 49% of the women agreed that having big breasts was a reason why women should get mammograms. Nearly one fifth of respondents (18%) believed that if they did not have a family history of breast cancer, they were unlikely to develop the disease, and close to two thirds (62%) of the women agreed that breastfeeding has a protective effect against breast cancer development.

The respondents reported more accurate perceptions on most of the other items in section 2 of the survey. For example, 92% of the women disagreed or strongly disagreed that women under 50 years of age did not need mammograms. This is particularly important given the relatively high incidence of breast cancer among women under age 35 reported in Thailand. Similar percentages of respondents agreed or strongly agreed that mothers should encourage their daughters to get mammograms when they reach 40 years of age and disagreed that healthy women do not need mammograms. Virtually all the women who responded (99%) agreed that early diagnosis promotes effective treatment.

The women in this study also reported some inaccurate perceptions of risks for and causes of breast cancer in section 5 of the survey tool. For example, trauma to breasts in any form was believed by 42% if the women to contribute to cancer, and 13% of the women believed that mammography itself could cause disease, similar to the response to the item included in section 2. The majority of the women (76% and 75%, respectively) believed that hormone replacement therapy and consumption of certain foods, such as high fat and oily food, beef, and grilled food, caused breast cancer. Fifty-eight percent of the participants agreed or strongly agreed that emotional stress could increase one's risk of breast cancer, and a number of participants (40%) perceived karma (fate) as a cause of breast cancer. Finally, a large proportion (85%) of the respondents believed that breast cancer might result from breast augmentation. Frequency distributions for responses for items related to perceptions of breast cancer, mammography, and causes of cancer are presented in Table 3.

Table 3. Percentage Distribution* of Responses to Items Related to Breast Cancer Perceptions

Perceptions of Breast Cancer and Mammography (Section 2)	SA	A	D	SD
1. Thai women rarely get breast cancer (N = 360)	9%	29%	31%	31%
2. Women who are younger than 50 don't need to get a mammogram (N = 360)	3%	5%	23%	69%
3. Women who are older than 70 don't need to get a mammogram (N = 360)	14%	22%	29%	36%
4. Mothers should tell their daughters to get a mammogram when they approach age 40 (N = 359)	75%	17%	4.5%	4%
5. Women who are healthy don't need to get a mammogram (N = 358)	4%	5%	18%	74%
6. It is not necessary to get a mammogram every year if that person has a normal mammogram (N = 358)	7.5%	12%	24%	56%
7. Women with small breasts rarely get breast cancer (N =359)	3%	10%	25%	62%
8. When the breast is traumatized by the mammogram device, it might cause cancer (N = 354)	2%	13%	28%	58%
9. You can get free mammograms (N = 360)	61%	13%	6%	19%
10. Finding out about breast cancer early makes it easier to cure (N = 359)	94%	5%	<1%	<1%
11. Women who are married are more likely to get breast cancer than women who are single (N = 359)	5%	16%	29%	50%

Perceptions of Breast Cancer and Mammography (Section 2)	SA	A	D	SD
12. Women who are not having sex are less likely to get breast cancer than those who have sex (N = 358)	4%	18%	32%	46%
13. If no one in your family has had breast cancer, you are not likely to get breast cancer (N = 360)	4%	14%	31%	51%
14. Breast feeding can help protect against cancer (N = 352)	20%	42%	23%	15%
Causes of Breast Cancer (Section 5)	**SA**	**A**	**D**	**SD**
1. Eating some types of food that cause cancer (N = 360)	33%	42%	16%	9%
2. Injury or trauma to their breasts (N = 358)	5%	37%	27%	30%
3. Squeezing or touching their breasts too much (N = 356)	2.5%	26%	30%	42%
4. Having a mammogram (N = 356)	2%	11%	26%	61%
5. Being a prostitute (N = 358)	7.5%	21%	31.5%	40%
6. Having sex (N = 358)	<1%	7%	20%	72%
7. Being married (N = 359)	<1%	4 %	19%	76%
8. Breast implants (N = 354)	41%	44%	11%	4.5%
9. Taking female hormones menopause symptoms (N = 357)	24%	52%	18%	6%
10. Emotional stress (N = 357)	20%	38%	26%	15%
11. Their karma (N = 357)	13%	27%	20%	39%

SA = Strongly Agree A = Agree D = Disagree SD = Strongly disagree
*Valid percent based on those responding. Percentages are rounded so may not total to 100%

Perceived factors promoting mammography participation. Section 3 of the survey tool addressed respondents' perceptions of factors that might motivate mammography participation. The participants agreed with a number of factors as promoting mammography screening. Recommendation from health care providers, for example, was perceived as strongly influencing screening participation. Ninety-one percent of the participants agreed or strongly agreed that provider recommendation was a motivator for screening participation.

Conversely, 30% of the women agreed that a provider recommendation against mammography would lead to nonparticipation. Both of these findings highlight the importance of provider recommendation in screening decisions and are consistent with the emphasis placed on provider recommendation by the focus group participants. Friends' or family's recommendation and exposure to media were perceived as promoting screening by 89% and 87% of the women, respectively.

Physical and psychological factors were also believed to influence screening behaviors. For example, the vast majority of the respondents agreed that Thai women would get a mammogram if they were worried about breast cancer (98%), were getting older and generally more health conscious (98%) , or were concerned about health in general (99%). Most of the women also agreed that finding a breast lump (97%), having a family history of breast cancer (97%), experiencing fluid leaking from their nipples (96%), taking HRT (93%), or having had breast implants (93%) were reasons that women would obtain a mammogram. Aging and menopause were also perceived as reasons for having a mammogram by 95% and 86% of the women, respectively. Frequency distributions for responses to items related to perceived motivators for mammography participation are presented in Table 4.

Perceived barriers to mammography participation. The women in this study perceived a variety of barriers to screening participation. Respondents agreed that factors related to screening services, such as lack of health insurance (82%) and cost of services (78%) were major barriers to mammography screening.

Pain related to the procedure or fear of pain was perceived by 33% and 37% of the women, respectively, as reasons for not getting a mammogram. More than half of the participants (52%), agreed that fear of finding cancer was an impediment to screening participation.

Distance to screening services was perceived by 46.5% of the participants as impeding screening. Furthermore, 40% of the women said that inconvenient days and times for mammography services were barriers to screening participation

In addition to inconvenience, the participants perceived that other responsibilities in their lives prevented Thai women from obtain screening. These included family responsibilities (31%) and inability to take time from work (23%). Overall, 28% of the women perceived a general lack of time as a factor in Thai women not obtaining mammograms. The percentages of women who perceived time issues as barriers to mammography were less than expected given the emphasis placed on these factors by women in the focus groups.

Table 4. Percentage Distribution* of Responses to Items Related to Factors Promoting Mammography Participation

Factors Promoting Mammography Participation (Section 3)	SA	A	D	SD
1. The doctor recommends it (N = 360)	69%	22%	5%	3%
2. They want to know if they have breast cancer so it can be treated early (N = 360)	84%	13%	3%	<1%
3. They are getting older and more conscious of health (N = 360)	67.5%	30.5%	2%	<1%
4. They are afraid of getting breast cancer, so they get the test to protect their health (N = 360)	83%	15%	2%	-
5. Friends or relatives suggest getting the test (N = 359)	46%	43%	6%	4.5%
6. They are concerned about health (N = 360)	64%	35%	1%	<1%
7. They learned from TV or advertising media that every woman should get the test (N = 360)	35%	52%	10%	3%
8. When they find a lump in their breasts (N = 360)	92%	5%	2%	2%
9. When they get older (N = 360)	68%	27%	2%	3%
10. When they stop having menstrual periods (N = 360)	66%	20%	5%	9%
11. When they are taking female hormones (N = 360)	76%	17%	5%	2%
12. When someone in their family has breast cancer (N = 360)	89%	8%	1%	2%
13. When they have big breasts (N = 360)	33%	16%	12%	39%
14. When water or fluid is leaking from their breasts (N = 360)	92%	4%	1%	2.5%
15. If they have had or currently have a breast implant (N = 357)	78%	15%	3%	3%

More than half of the women (53.5%) agreed that low perceptions of risk for breast cancer were a reason why Thai women might not obtain screening. Similarly, 45% of the respondents agreed that lack of perceived importance of screening was a factor that impeded mammography participation. Other perceived barriers to screening included cultural issues such as language difficulties, with which 68% of the women agreed, and reticence to expose their breasts perceived by 50% of the respondents. Frequency distributions for responses to items related to perceived barriers to mammography participation are presented in Table 5.

Table 5. Percentage Distribution* of Responses to Items Related to Factors Impeding Mammography Participation

Factors Impeding Mammography Participation (Section 4)	SA	A	D	SD
1. Based on past experience, it hurts (N = 356)	11%	22%	20%	47%
2. They don't want to know or are afraid of knowing if they have cancer (N = 360)	16%	32%	25.5%	22%
3. They don't have time to get checked because they have to take care of their families (N = 359)	4%	27%	27%	42%
4. They can't take time from work (N = 360)	3%	20%	29%	48%
5. They are shy about having their breasts checked (N = 360)	19%	31%	18%	32%
6. The days and times for mammograms are not convenient (N = 359)	5%	35%	27.5%	32.5%
7. Hospitals or places where mammograms are done are far from home (N = 360)	7.5%	39%	27%	27%
8. They have to pay for the service (N = 360)	44%	34%	10%	12%
9. They don't have health insurance (N = 360)	50%	32%	9%	8%
10. They don't have anyone to go with them; they don't feel comfortable going alone (N = 360)	9%	42.5%	24%	24%
11. They cannot speak English and don't understand it; they need an interpreter (N = 360)	21%	47%	18%	14%
12. The doctor said they don't need a mammogram (N = 360)	8%	22%	43%	27.5%

Factors Impeding Mammography Participation (Section 4)	SA	A	D	SD
13. They don't think they will get cancer, so there is no need for the test (N = 360)	20.5%	33%	17%	29%
14. They don't think it is important (N = 360)	16%	29%	19%	35.5%
15. They don't have time (N = 360)	6%	22%	31%	41%
16. They are afraid the test will be pianful (N = 360)	9%	28%	23%	40%

SA = Strongly Agree A = Agree D = Disagree SD = Strongly disagree

*Valid percent based on those responding. Percentages are rounded so may not total to 100%

Relationship of Influencing Factors to Mammography Participation. Statistically significant differences in mammography participation were noted for women of different ages (*z* score -5.777, p. < .001). Women 51 to 60 years of age were more likely to have had a mammogram than either younger or older women. Similarly, there were significant differences in mammography participation based on length of time in the United States (z = -6.809, p. < .001)

Not surprisingly, women with a consistent provider were significantly more likely than those without to have ever had a mammogram (x^2 = 15.67, p. < .001). Similarly women with health insurance were more likely to have ever had a mammogram (x^2 = 17.18, p. < .001) than those without insurance.

Table 6 presents the results of Mann Whitney U tests of differences between women who had ever had a mammogram and those who had never had one with respect to selected influencing factors. As noted in the table, there were highly significant differences (p. < .001) between the two groups with respect to perceptions that one does not need regular mammography after a negative test result and awareness of free mammography services. Women who had never had a mammogram were more likely to believe that a prior negative mammogram precluded the need for subsequent screening. Not surprisingly, these women were also less likely to be aware of free or low-cost mammography services in the community.

Women who had not mammograms were more likely than those who had to agree that healthy women did not need mammograms and that mammograms were painful (p < .01). In addition, these women were more significantly likely to perceive inconvenient times for services and language barriers as impediments to obtaining a mammogram (p < .01).

Moderately significant differences (p. < .05) were noted between women who had ever had and never had mammograms for perceptions related to the influence of age on the need for mammography and perceptions that HRT and mammography itself might cause breast cancer. Women who reported never having a mammogram were more likely than their screened counterparts to agree both that women less than 50 years of age and those over 70 years of age did not need mammograms. Similarly, those without a history of mammography participation were more likely to perceive HRT and mammography participation as causes of cancer.

There were no significant differences between the two groups regarding their perception of Thai women's risk for breast cancer, the influence of health provider recommendations not to get a mammogram, or lack of time as a deterrent to screening. The latter finding is surprising given the emphasis placed on lack of time for screening by focus group participants in the prior study.

Table 6. Mann-Whitney *U* Tests of Differences Between Women Who Ever Had and Never Had a Mammogram on Selected Factors

Factor	z	p
Perceptions of low breast cancer risk for Thai women	-.962	NS
Women < 50 do not need mammograms	-2.233	< .05
Women > 70 do not need mammograms	-2.183	< .05
Healthy women do not need mammograms	-2.802	< .01
Previous negative mammogram preclude need for futher screening	-3.888	< .001
Mammogram causes breast cancer	-2.219	< .05
HRT causes breast cancer	-2.247	< .05
Knowledge of free services	-3.892	< .001
Health provider recommenation not to get a mammogram	-1.472	NS
Perception of mammogram as painful	-2.791	< .01
Lack of time	-0.722	NS
Inconvenient times for services	-2.691	< .01
Language barrier as impediment	-3.258	< .01

NS = Non-significant

Relationship of influencing factors to mammography frequency. No differences were noted among various age groups with respect to receiving annual mammography or mammography less often than every three years (U = 3675.5, p = .378). Frequency of mammography participation was, however, statistically significantly related to time in residence in the United States, with women who had been here fewer than five years being more likely to get mammograms at intervals greater than three years (U = 3280, p = .004). Not surprisingly, women without regular health care providers were more likely have more than three years between mammograms than those with regular providers (x^2 = 21/325, p < .001). With respect to insurance status, results were again as might be expected. Women without health insurance were more likely to experience mammography less often than every three years (x^2 = 17.962, p. < .001).

Table 7 presents the results of t-tests of differences between women who had annual mammograms and those who had mammograms less often than every three years with regard to selected factors believed to influence participation. As indicated in Table 7, no highly significant differences (p < .001) were noted between the two groups. A moderately significant difference (p .01) in the expected direction was noted for agreement with provider recommendation against mammography as a deterrent to screening, with women reporting less frequent mammography participation more likely to agree with this statement. A similar finding was noted for respondent's perceptions that older women do not need mammograms.

Less significant differences (p .05) were noted for perceptions of low breast cancer risk for Thai women, mammography as a cause of breast cancer, and lack of time as a deterrent to mammography participation. Women who reported histories of mammograms less often than every three years were more likely than those reporting annual mammograms to agree that Thai women rarely get breast cancer and that having a mammogram might actually cause cancer. They were also more likely to agree that lack of time impedes mammography participation. Another mildly significant difference (p .05) was noted between the groups with respect to years spent in the United States, with less time in residence linked to less frequent mammography. Nonsignificant differences were noted between women with annual mammograms and those with less frequent mammograms with respect to perceptions of HRT as a cause of cancer, views of mammography as painful, or perceptions of language barriers as an impediment to screening.

Table 7. T-tests for Differences Between Women Reporting Annual Mammograms and Those Reporting a Frequency Greater Than Every Three Years on Selected Factors,

Factor	t	p
Years in the United States	2.565*	.05
Perceptions of low breast cancer risk for Thai women	2.086	< .05
Women < 50 do not need mammograms	NC	NC
Women > 70 do not need mammograms	2.748*	.01
Healthy women do not need mammograms	NC	NC
Previous negative mammogram preclude need for futher screening	NC	NC
Mammogram causes breast cancer	2.438*	.05
HRT causes breast cancer	.000	NS
Knowledge of free services	NC	NC
Health provider recommenation not to get a mammogram	-3.066	.01
Perception of mammogram as painful	-.612	NS
Lack of time	-2.357	.05
Inconvenient times for services	NC	NC
Lack of health insurance	-4.138*	.001
Language barrier as impediment	-1.657	NS

* Without assumption of equal variance

NC = Statistic not calculated due to lack of variation in percentage of responses between groups

NS = Non-significant

Spearman rho correlations among influencing factors, frequency of mammography, and intentions to obtain a mammogram in the coming year are presented in Table 8. Higher scores for the accuracy of perceptions related to breast cancer and breast cancer screening were not significantly correlated with mammography frequency, but achieved a moderately significant positive correlation (p .01) with intentions to obtain a mammogram in the next year. Years in the United States was correlated with both mammography frequency and screening intentions with longer residence associated with annual mammography and with greater intentions to be screened. Being acquainted with other Thai women with diagnoses of breast cancer was moderately positively correlated with mammography frequency (p .01), and slightly less so with screening intentions (p .05). Conversely, agreement that healthy women do not need mammograms was negatively correlated with mammography frequency. Increasing age was mildly (p.05) positively correlated with future intentions, but was not associated with frequency. Finally, mammography frequency correlated with screening intentions (p. 01) in the expected direction.

Table 8. Spearman Rho Correlations among Perceptions of Selected Influencing Factors, Mammography Frequency and Future Intentions for Screening Participation

Influencing Factor	Mammography Frequency		Screening Intentions	
	r_s	p	r_s	p
More accurate perceptions score	0.104	NS	0.327	.01
Increasing age	0.062	NS	0.116	.05
Years in the United States	0.193	.01	0.160	.01
Health insurance	0.293	.01	0.184	.01
Belief in HRT as a cause of breast cancer	0.011	NS	NC	NC
Acquainted with Thai women with BCA	0.269	.01	0.153	.05
Healthy women don't need mammograms	-0.169	.01	NC	NC
Lack of time	-0.129	.05	NC	NC
Frequency of mammograms			0.520	.01

NC = Statistic not calculated due to lack of variation in percentage of responses
NS = Non-significant

Interactions among influencing factors. Interactions were also noted between some of the influencing factors addressed in this study. Not surprisingly, having health insurance was significantly positively associated with having a regular health care provider. In addition, higher scores for accuracy of perceptions were significantly inversely correlated with age, with younger women exhibiting higher scores (r_s = 0.161, p. 0.01). Age also influenced perceptions regarding the salience of several influencing factors. Belief in karma as a cause of cancer, for example, was significantly correlated with increasing age (r_s = 0.142, p. 0.01). Younger women, on the other hand, were more likely than older respondents to disagree that prostitution causes breast cancer, but older women were more likely to disagree with mammography as a cause of cancer (r_s = -0.165, p. 0.01, r_s = 0.107, p. 0.05)

Discussion

This study explored mammography screening behaviors and factors contributing to screening among Thai-American women 40 years of age and over in southern California. The current U.S. Preventive Services Task Force guidelines for mammography screening are for biennial screening for women 50 to 74 years of age with earlier and later screening to be determined on an individual basis with consideration of the patient context (USPSTF, 2009a). The American Cancer Society (2010), Susan G. Komen for the Cure (2010), and the Memorial Sloan-Kettering Cancer Center (2008), on the other hand, continue to recommend annual screening for women over 40 years of age, continuing as long as the woman is in good health. The American College of Obstetricians and Gynecologists (2006) has promulgated similar recommendations except that women from 40 to 49 years of age should be screened every 1 to 2 years.

A systematic review of repeat mammography (Clark, Rakowski, & Bonacore, 2003) found that less than half (46%) of women from all ethnic groups receive mammograms regularly. In this study, 59% of Thai women living in southern California reported obtaining a mammogram in the prior year, consistent with data reported by the Thai Community Development Center in 2004, but less than the 65% of API women in the United States and even farther below the 70% target established for all U.S. women (CDC, 2010). However, 16% of the women in the current study had never had a mammogram and another 16% received mammograms less often than every three years, indicating a need for further effort to promote screening participation.

Although younger women in this study had more accurate perceptions of breast cancer, mammography use was more prevalent among women 51-60 years of age. Women over age 50 were also more likely to indicate intentions to participate in screening in the coming year. Comparative figures, however, suggest that Thai women develop breast cancer at younger ages than U.S. women. For example, in 2004 the incidence of invasive breast cancer in U.S. women under 50 years of age was 43.5 per 100,000 women versus 335.7 in women over 50 (National Cancer Institute, NIH, 2007). In Thailand, however, women under age 50 accounted for 52% of all breast cancer cases diagnosed in 2006 (National Cancer Institute, MOPH, 2006)

The findings of this study indicate that more than a third of the Thai women participating believed they have a low breast cancer risk, similar to findings among Chinese-American women (Facione, Giancarlo, & Chan, 2000). This low perception of risk may be impeding effective breast cancer screening, and education should seek to change these perceptions

Recommendations from health care providers and friends were seen as major positive influences on mammography screening in this population. This is consistent with findings related to the general U.S. population as well as other ethnic groups (Fernandez, Palmer, & Leong-Wu, 2005). Lack of health insurance and not having a regular health care provider were perceived by focus group members as major reasons why Thai women in southern California might not participate in screening programs. These perceptions were supported by the differences in reported screening participation based on health insurance status and having a regular provider found in this study. Similar to women in other minority groups, large numbers of Thai women living in southern California were without health insurance. Language difficulty was another perceived reason for not receiving a mammogram, a finding consistent with studies in other ethnic groups such as Chinese, Korean, Filipino, and Asian Indian American women (Wu et al., 2005), Japanese American women (Sadler et al., 2001), and Thai women (Clark & Natipagon-Shah, 2008).

The finding that 92% of the women stated they would or might get a mammogram in the coming year is interesting since it exceeds the percentage of women in the population who had ever had a mammogram and particularly exceeds the percentage of those who reported annual mammograms. There are two possible explanations for this finding. First, it may be a function of response bias, with respondents providing the response they believe is expected by the interviewers. The second possibility is that participation in the study served as a cue to action motivating at least contemplation of obtaining a mammogram in the next year.

In this study, years living in the United States was viewed as a marker for acculturation. Longer residence was significantly associated with greater mammography use, frequency of mammography, and intent to obtain a mammogram in the next year This is consistent with findings by Pineda and associates (2001) that acculturation is not associated with decreased breast cancer survival in API women and suggests that interventions to promote screening should be particularly targeted to recent immigrants.

Limitations

The findings of this study are limited by the self-reported nature of the data, which may have been compounded by a cultural tendency to give others the information one thinks is desired. Relatively few women refused to participate in the study even after being informed of its voluntary nature. This may be another reflection of expectations of courtesy operating in Thai culture. Limitations also arise from the relatively small sample size and from the use of telephone interviews, which may not allow participants to fully consider their responses.

Use of an investigator-developed tool may also be a limitation. However, the tool was grounded in the findings of prior research with this population and was reviewed with members of the target population to assure cultural and linguistic appropriateness. In addition, pilot tests of the tool indicated its utility. The phrasing of some questions and response options would undoubtedly be modified if the study were to be repeated.

In addition, the use of snowball sampling might have resulted in a highly homogenous sample. However, the variability on such items as age, years in the United States, presence or absence of a regular health care provider, and insurance status suggests that this was not the case.

Conclusion

A number of factors appear to be perceived as negatively influencing mammography screening participation among Thai women living in southern California. Chief among these are perceptions of low breast cancer risk, a variety of misperceptions about breast cancer and mammography screening, younger age, and recent arrival in the United States. Lack of a regular provider and health insurance were other deterrents to screening participation, but could be offset by better dissemination of information about free or low-cost mammography services. Finally, language difficulties often impeded mammography participation.

These findings suggest that interventions should be directed toward correcting misperceptions regarding cancer risk, planning for linguistically and culturally appropriate services at times convenient to the population, and increasing knowledge of the availability of mammography services. In addition, these interventions should be particularly targeted to Thai women less than 50 years of age and to recent immigrants. Given the importance of provider recommendations in promoting screening, health care providers serving the Thai population should also be encouraged to regularly discuss screening needs with their clients. There is a need to develop and test interventions for improving mammography participation among certain subgroups within the southern California Thai population.

REFERENCES

Altekruse, S.F., Kosary, C.L., Krapcho, M., Neyman, N., Aminou. R., Waldron, W., . . Edwards, B.K. (Eds). (2010). *SEER Cancer Statistics Review, 1975-2007* (Table 4.19). Retrieved January 13, 2011 from http://seer.cancer.gov

American Cancer Society. (2009). *Breast cancer facts & figures, 2009-2010.* Retrieved January 13, 2011 from http://www.cancer.com

American Cancer Society. (2010). *American Cancer Society Guidelines for the early detection of cancer.* Retrieved January 21, 2011 from http://www.cancer.org/Healthy/FindCancerEarly/CancerScreeningGuidelines/american-cancer-society-guidelines-for-the-early-detection-of-cancer

American College of Obstetricians and Gynecologists. (2006). *Breast Cancer Screening.* Retrieved January 21, 2011 from http://www.guideline.gov/content.aspx?id=3990#Section420

Avci, I. A., & Kurt, H. (2008). Health beliefs and mammography rates of Turkish women living in rural areas. *Journal of Nursing Scholarship, 40,* 170-175.

Brooks, P., Hamilton, J., & Powe, B. (2006). Perceptions of cancer fatalism and cancer knowledge: A comparison of older and younger African American women. *Journal of Psychosocial Oncology, 24,* 1-13.

Burgess, C. C., Linsell, L., & Ramirez, A. J. (2008). Breast cancer awareness among older women. *British Journal of Cancer, 99,* 1221-1225.

Centers for Disease Control and Prevention. (2010). *Data 2010: The Healthy People 2010 database.* Retrieved January 13, 2011 from http://wonder.cdc.gov/data2010

Choi, K. S., Lee, S., Park, E.-C., Kwak, M.-S., Spring, B. J., & Juon, H.-S. (2010). Comparison of breast cancer screening rates between Korean women in America versus Korea. *Journal of Women's Health, 19,* 1089-1096. doi: 10.1089/jwh.2009.1584

Clark, M. A., Rakowski, W., & Bonacore, L. B. (2003). Repeat mammography: Prevalence estimates and considerations for assessment. *Annals of Behavioral Medicine, 26*, 201–11.

Clark, M. J., & Natipagon-Shah, B. (2008). Thai American women's perceptions regarding mammography participation. *Public Health Nursing, 25*, 212-220.

Daddario, D. K. (2007). A review of the use of the Health Belief Model for weight management. *MEDSURG Nursing, 16*, 363-366.

Eremenco, S. L., Cella, D., & Arnold, B. J. (2005). A comprehensive method for the translation and cross-cultural validation of health status questionnaires. *Evaluation and the Health Professions, 28*, 212-232. doi: 28/2/212 [pii]10.1177/0163278705275342

Facione, N., Giancarlo, C., & Chan, L. (2000). Perceived risk and help-seeking behavior for breast cancer: A Chinese-American perspective. *Cancer Nursing, 23*, 258-267.

Fernandez, M. E., Palmer, R. C., & Leong-Wu, C. A. (2005). Repeat mammography screening among low-income and minority women: A qualitative study. *Cancer Control: Journal of the Moffitt Cancer Center, 12*(Suppl. 2), 77-83.

Garza, M. A., Luna, J., Blinka, M., Farabee-Lewis, Neuhaus, C. E., Zabora, J. R., & Ford, J. G. (2005). A culturally targeted intervention to promote breast cancer screening among low-income women in East Baltimore, Maryland. *Cancer Control: Journal of the Moffitt Cancer Center, 12*(Suppl. 2), 34-41.

Gatewood, J. G., Litchfield, R. E., Ryan, S. J., Geadalmann, J. D. M., Pendergast, J. F., & Ullom, K. K. (2008). Perceived barriers to community-based health program participation. *American Journal of Health Behavior, 32*, 260-271.

Gilani, G. M., & Kamal, S., (2004). Risk factors for breast cancer in Pakastani women aged less than 45 years. *Annals of Human Biology, 31*, 398-407.

Glenn, B. A., Chawla, N., Surani, Z., & Bastani, R. (2009). Rates and sociodemographic correlates of cancer screening among South Asians. *Journal of Community Health, 34*, 113-121. doi: 10.1007/s10900-008-9129-1

Green, L. W. (1974). Forward. In M. H. Becker (Ed.), *The Health Belief Model and personal health behavior* (p. iii). Thoroughfare, NJ: Charles B. Slack.

Groenewald, T. (2004). A phenomenological research design illustrated. *International Journal of Qualitative Methods, 3*(1). Article 4. Retrieved January 14, 2011 from http://ejournals.library.ualberta.ca/index.php/IJQM/article/view/4484/3622

Guilfoyle, S., Franco, R., & Gorin, S. S. (2007). Exploring older women's approaches to cervical cancer screening. *Health Care for Women International, 28*, 930-950.

Ham, O. K. (2007). The intention of future mammography screening among Korean women. *Journal of Community Health Nursing, 22*(1), 1-13.

International Agency for Research on Cancer. (2008). *Globocan 2008 fast stats: Thailand.* Retrieved January 13, 2011 from http://globocan.iarc.fr/factsheets/populations/factsheet.asp?uno=764

Jordan, S., Lim, L., Vilainerun, D., Banks. E., Sripaiboonk, N., Seubsman, S., . . . Bain, C. (2009). Breast cancer in the Thai cohort study: An exploratory case-control analysis. *Breast* (Edinbourgh, Scottland), *18*(5-3), 299-303.

Ka`opua, L. S., & Anngela, L. (2005). Developing a spiritually based breast cancer screening intervention for Native Hawaiian women. *Cancer Control: Journal of the Moffitt Cancer Center, 12*(Suppl. 2), 97-99.

Kumsuk, S. (2005). *Breast cancer beliefs and mammography screening among Thai-American women.* Retrieved January 13, 2011 from http://www.apha.confex.com/apha/133am/techprogram/paper_103277.htm

Kumsuk, S. (2006). *An understanding of breast cancer beliefs and mammography use among Thai women in the United States* (Unpublished doctoral dissertation). Saint Louis University, St. Louis, MO.

Lee, H., Kim, J., & Han, H.-R. (2009). Do cultural factors predict mammography behavior among Korean immigrants in the USA? *Journal of Advanced Nursing, 65*, 2574-2584. doi: 10.1111/j.1365-2648.2009.05155.x

Lee-Lin, F., Menon, U., Pett, M., Nail, L., Lee, S., & Mooney, K. (2007). Breast cancer beliefs and mammography screening practices among Chinese American immigrants. *JOGNN, 36*, 212-221.

Ma, G. X., Shive, S. E., Wang, M. Q., & Tan, Y. (2009). Cancer screening behaviors and barriers in Asian Americans. *American Journal of Health Behavior, 33*, 650-660.

Martin, N., & Patel, N. (2003). Cancer incidence and leading sites. In H. Sriplung, S. Sontipong, M. Martin, S. Wiangnan, V. Votriprux, A. Chearsilpa, et al. (Eds.), *Cancer in Thailand* (pp. 9-18). Retrieved January 18, 2011 from http://www.nci.go.th/file_download/Cancer%20In%20Thailand/CHARTER2.pdf

Memorial Sloan-Kettering Cancer Center. (2008). *Breast cancer screening guidelines*. Retrieved January 21, 2011 from http://www.mskcc.org/mskcc/html/65280.cfm#282973

Menon, U., Champion, V., Monahan, P. O., Daggy, J., Hui, S., & Skinner, C. S. (2007). Health Belief Model variables as predictors of progression in stage of mammography adoption. *American Journal of Health Promotion, 21,* 255-261.

Ministry of Public Health. (n.d.a). *Thailand health profile, 2001-2004.* Retrieved December 23, 2007 from http://www.moph.go.th/ops/health_48

Ministry of Public Health, Thailand. (n.d.b). *Thailand health profile, 2005-2007* (in Thai). Retrieved January 16, 2011 from http://www.moph.go.th/ops/thp/index.php?option=com_content&task=view&id=6&Itemid=2

National Cancer Institute, National Institutes of Health. (n.d.). *Stage distribution (SEER summary stage 2000) by race/ethnicity: Female breast, all ages, female, 2000-2007* Retrieved January 18, 2011 from http://www.seer.cancer

National Cancer Institute, National Institutes of Health. (2007). *Female breast cancer (invasive), Age-adjusted SEER incidence rates by year, race, and age.* Retrieved January 2, 2008 from http://seer.cancer

National Cancer Institute, National Institutes of Health. (2010). *SEER Stat fact sheets: Breast cancer.* Retrieved January 13, 2011 from http://seer.cancer.gov/statfacts/html/breast.html

National Cancer Institute, Ministry of Public Health, Thailand. (2006). *Cancer registry 2006.* Retrieved December 23, 2007 from http://www.nci.go.th/file-download/nci%20Cancer%20Registry/Cancer20.pdf

National Center for Chronic Disease Prevention and Health Promotion. (2009). *BRFFS: Chronic disease indicators*. Retrieved January 13, 2011 from http://apps.nccd.cdc.gov/cdi/SearchResults.aspx?IndicatorIds=76,73,59,57,45,51,63,70,58,53,47,41,65,69,72,75,48,42,23,18,27,25,13,20&StateIds=46&StateNames=United%20States&FromPage=HomePage

Palmer, R. C., Fernandez, M. E., Tortolero-Luna, G., Gonzales, A., & Mullen, P. D. (2005). Acculturation and mammography screening among Hispanic women living in farmworker communities. *Cancer Control: Journal of the Moffitt Cancer Center, 12*(Sippl. 2), 21-27.

Phipps, E., Cohen, M. H., Sorn, R., & Braitman, L. E. (1999). A pilot study of cancer knowledge and screening behaviors of Vietnamese and Cambodian women. *Health Care for Women International, 20*, 195-207.

Pineda, M. D., White, E., Kristal, A. R., & Taylor, V. (2001). Asian breast cancer survival in the US: A comparison between Asian immigrants, US-born Asian Americans and Caucasians. *International Journal of Epidemiology, 30*, 976-982.

Powe, B. D. (1995). Cancer fatalism among elderly Caucasians and African Americans. *Oncology Nursing, 26,* 1355-1359.

Putthasri, W., Tangcharoensathien, V., Mugem, S., & Jindawatana, W. (2004). Geographical distribution and utilization of mammography in Thailand. *Regional Health Forum, 8*(1), 84-91.

Rosenstock, I. M. (1974). The origins of the Health Belief Model. In M. H. Becker (Ed.), *The Health Belief Model and personal health behavior* (pp. 1-8). Thoroughfare, NJ: Charles B. Slack.

Sadler, G. R., Dhanjal, S. K., Shah, N. B., Ko, C., Anghel, M., & Harshburger, R. (2001). Asian Indian women: Knowledge, attitudes, and behaviors toward early breast cancer detection. *Public Health Nursing, 18*, 357-363. doi: 10.1046/j.1525-1446.2001.00357.x

Sadler, G. R., Takahashi, M., Ko, C. M., & Nguyen, T. (2003). Japanese American women: Behaviors and attitudes toward breast cancer education and screening. *Health Care for Women International, 24*, 18-26.

Sassi, F., Luft, H. S., & Guadagnoli, E. (2006). Reducing racial/ethnic disparities in female breast cancer: Screening rates and stage at diagnosis. *American Journal of Public Health, 96,* 2165-2172.

Smith, R. A., Cokkinides, V., & Eyre, H. J. (2005). American Cancer Society guidelines for the early detection of cancer, 2005. *CA: A Cancer Journal for Clinicians, 55*, 31–44.

Somanchi, M., Juon, H.-S., Rimal, R. (2010). Predictors of screening mammography among Asian Indian American women: A cross-sectional study in the Baltimore-Washington metropolitan area. *Journal of Women's Health, 19*, 433-441. doi:10.1089/jwh.2008.0873

Su, X., Ma, G. X., Seals, B., Tan, Y., & Hausman, A. (2006). Breast cancer early detection among Chinese women in the Philadelphia area. *Journal of Women's Health, 15*, 507-519.

Susan G. Komen for the Cure. (2010). *Early screening and detection.* Retrieved January 21, 2011 fromhttp://ww5.komen.org/Breast Cancer/GeneralRecommendations.html

Thai Community Development Center. (2004). *Healthcare on the margins: The precarious state of physical health for Thais in Thai Town*. Los Angeles: Author.

Thongsuksai, P., Chongsuvivatwong, V., & Sriplung, H. (2000). Delay in breast cancer care: A study in Thai women. *Medical Care, 38*(1), 108-114.

U. S. Census Bureau. (2000). *People born in Thailand.* Retrieved January 13, 2011 from http://www.census.gov/population/cen2000/stp-159/STP-159-thailand.pdf

U.S. Preventive Services Task Force. (2009a). Screening for Breast Cancer. Retrieved January 21, 2011 from http://www.uspreventiveservicestaskforce.org/uspstf/uspsbrca.htm

U. S. Preventive Services Task Force. (2009b). *Screening for Breast Cancer: Systematic Evidence Review Update for the U. S. Preventive Services Task Force* (AHRQ Publication No. 10-05142-EF-1).. Retrieved from http://www.uspreventiveservicestaskforce.org/uspstf09/breastcancer/brcanes.pdf

Vatanasapt, V., Sriamporn, S., & Vatanasapt, P. (2002). Cancer control in Thailand. *Japanese Journal of Clinical Oncology, 32*(Supplement 1), S82-S91.

Wilailak, S. (2009). Epidemiologic report of gynecologic cancer in Thailand. *Journal of Gynecological Oncology, 20*(2), 81-83. doi: 10.3802/jgo.2009.20.2.81

Wu, T.-Y., & Bancroft, J. (2006). Filipino American women's perceptions and experiences with breast cancer screening. *Oncology Nursing Forum, 33*, E71-E78. doi: 10.1188/06.ONF.E71-E78

Wu, T.-Y., Bancroft, J., & Guthrie, B. (2005). An integrative review on breast cancer screening practice and correlates among Chinese, Korean, Filipino, and Asian Indian American women. *Health Care for Women International, 26*, 225-246.

Wu, T.-Y., & Ronis, D. (2009). Correlates of recent and regular mammography screening among Asian-American Women. *Journal of Advanced Nursing, 65*, 2434-2446. doi: 10.1111/j.1365-2648.2009.05112.x

Yu., M., Seetoo, A. D., Hong, O. S., Song, L., Raizade, R., & Weller, A. L. A. (2002). Cancer screening promotion among medically underserved Asian American women: Integration of research and practice. *Research & Theory for Nursing Practice, 16*, 237-262.

In: Mammography:
Editors: A. Palmetti, R. Roux
ISBN 978-1-61470-589-5

Chapter 2

DIGITAL BREAST TOMOSYNTHESIS

***Luís Janeiro*[1,2], *Nuno Matela*[1], *Nuno Oliveira*[1] and *Pedro Almeida*[1]**

[1] Universidade de Lisboa, Faculdade de Ciências, Instituto de Biofísica e Engenharia Biomédica, Lisbon, Portugal

[2] Escola Superior de Saúde da Cruz Vermelha, Portugal

ABSTRACT

Digital breast tomosynthesis (DBT) is an emerging radiological technique that can be used for breast cancer imaging. It produces a three-dimensional image from a series of projections or views, reducing the problem of overlapping structures and consequently allowing depth localisation of lesions, better discrimination of tissues and an overall better contrast. These advantages may allow a diagnosis with higher sensitivity and lower number of false positives and can pave the way for DBT as an alternative to planar mammography in breast cancer screening, particularly for women with dense breasts

Technically, tomosynthesis equipment is similar to digital mammography equipment. The main difference lies in the possibility of acquiring projections in different angular positions. To prevent an increase of the absorbed dose by the patient, the acquisition time in each position is substantially lower when compared to the one of a mammogram. The choice of the acquisition parameters is still a matter of study and different manufacturers suggested different numbers of projections and different angular range. These differences reflect in the thickness of the reconstructed volume slices and in the examination time, which will impact on patient comfort and possible artifacts related to motion.

Each projection individually does not have clinical value due to the low number of x-rays detected. Thus, the set of projections must be reconstructed, resulting in a 3D image volume that can be visualised in slices with typically 1 mm thickness. Initial tomosynthesis experiments made use of simple reconstruction algorithms such as the shift-and-add algorithm. Iterative algorithms for tomosynthesis image reconstruction are being investigated and they were found to be superior to analytical algorithms for masses and small calcifications detection. These algorithms have a common root with the ones used in nuclear medicine because they are suitable for situations with low acquisition statistics. The usage of these algorithms may permit an improvement in image quality or alternatively a reduction in exposure time, maintaining an image quality similar to that is currently provided.

Although the concept of tomosynthesis has long been known, its application in diagnosis of breast cancer is relatively recent and has not received yet approval from the FDA (Food and Drug Administration) for its use in the US. The leading manufacturers grant access to some equipment to some research groups and hospitals to conduct the first clinical trials and results indicate that screening examinations performed with tomosynthesis and mammography together can be reduced by approximately 40% the number of people recalled for reassessment, thus confirming a reduction in the number of false positives. The results of these trials seem to indicate also that tomosynthesis may have an important role not only as a supplementary examination after mammography screening, but also in cases of follow-up and diagnosis of symptomatic patients.

Introduction

X-ray mammography (both digital and film-screen) is considered the most effective imaging modality for detecting the early stages of breast cancer. However, it can not separately identify overlying tissue, which results in anatomical noise. This kind of noise is one of the biggest obstacles to the interpretation of mammograms and results in a considerable number of wrong diagnoses. Breast tomosynthesis emerged as a refinement of digital mammography, attempting to overcome this limitation by acquiring several projection images at different angular positions around a fixed point close to the centre of the detector. Series of 2D slice images of the breast are then reconstructed from these projections [1]. However, the number of projections acquired is limited by the total dose which should be comparable to that used in conventional mammography. Commercial versions of tomosynthesis systems for breast imaging are now very close to market approval.

X-RAY DETECTION

This section will start by an explanation of the technology behind the detection of the x-rays in tomosynthesis scanners. After this, we will discuss the different acquisition sequences that are currently considered by the manufacturers and the consequences of these options on image quality, examination length and absorbed dose. Finally we will present some of the new developments related with the acquisition that are currently being tested to be introduced in the market.

Digital acquisition technology

The x-ray detection in tomosynthesis can be performed with Cesium iodide crystal detectors or with amorphous selenium detectors. Amorphous selenium technology seems to be the most appropriate technology due to its high efficiency when detecting x-rays with energies suitable for breast imaging. When x-rays are absorber by amorphous selenium, electric charges are released as electron-hole pairs. By applying an electric field with two electrodes to both extremities of the detector, these charges can be pulled by electrode pads and collected without the need of any indirect conversion of light in an electrical signal [2]. In addition to its higher efficiency, this kind of detectors also present high modulation transfer function.

This kind of detector has already been fully characterised for its usage in breast tomosynthesis [3]. The results proved its high modulation transfer function and lower noise levels and also confirm it has suitable temporal performance, allowing high frame rates as it is required in tomosynthesis.

Acquisition procedure

To overcome the limitation of overlapping tissues, in tomosynthesis the radiation is acquired in several angular projections. To do this, one uses a moving x-ray source and a movable or unmovable digital detector, which is normally possible with minor modifications to a digital mammograph.

The x-ray tube movement can be linear, circular or even elliptic around the breast. However the most common configuration corresponds to a motion along an arc around an unmovable detector. In this case, the centre of rotation is a point close to detector surface (Figure 1).

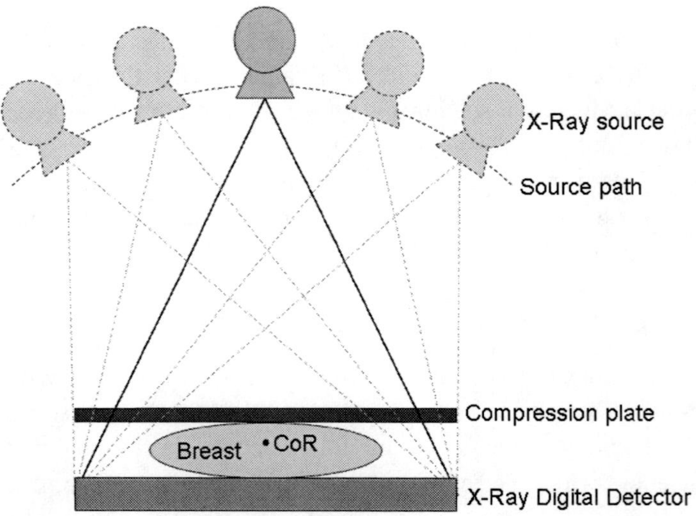

Figure 1. Acquisition scheme of a tomosynthesis examination. An x-ray source irradiates the breast in different angular positions. CoR stands for centre of rotation.

One of the biggest worries regarding the use of tomosynthesis is the reduction of dose absorbed by the patients. As in digital mammography, the absorbed dose is proportional to the total exposure time. Trying to keep tomosynthesis dose at acceptable limits, the manufacturers established that the total dose of a tomosynthesis examination should not exceed the dose of two digital mammograms, which corresponds to a common breast examination. Having this assumption, increasing the number of projections leads to a decrease in the exposure time per projection, resulting in noisier images, despite introducing more information. Because of this, the angular range and the number of projections are not consensual between different manufacturers and many studies have been published addressing this issue.

One of the most complete studies in this context was performed by Sechopoulos and Ghetti [4]. In this study, 63 combinations of angular ranges and number of projections were evaluated by computer simulations. These different combinations were compared regarding how they affect the quality of image reconstruction, lesion visibility, vertical spatial resolution, contrast-to-noise ratio and artifact spread function. As expected, increasing angular coverage increases vertical resolution. However, after reaching a certain threshold, increasing the number of projections has no additional effect on vertical resolution. The value of this threshold was found to be proportional to the angular range, which means that larger angular coverage requires a larger number of projections. A similar conclusion was found when analysing the artifact spread function. One of the assumptions of this study was that the total exposure should be kept constant in all combinations. This led to projections with higher noise levels when a larger number of projections were considered resulting in an inverse relationship between contrast-to-noise ratio and the number of projections. However, the benefit in vertical resolution observed with larger angular coverage results in higher contrast-to-noise ratio values. After comparing all combinations, the authors concluded that the best results were obtained with 13 projections over a 60° angular coverage.

Zhao *et al.* in [5] also concluded that larger angular coverage produces images with higher quality regarding noise and modulation transfer function values. Besides this, Zhao *et al.* also evaluated the possibility of using the detector not in a full resolution mode but with 2x1 pixel binning. This procedure would reduce the acquisition time, maintaining noise levels. If the acquisition time is maintained, acquiring in the binning mode allows lower noise levels and better masses detection. In other study [3] the same authors showed that pixel binning has a higher effect on modulation transfer function than focal spot blurring due to the tube movement. The authors also evaluated two characteristics that are extremely important for rapid image acquisitions which are lag and ghosting. Lag corresponds to the residues of image charges induced by previous exposures of the detector and ghosting corresponds to changes in detector sensitivity due to repeated exposures. The results show a lag of 8% from the first frame with the detector working in a 2x1 binning mode and a lag of 4% in the full resolution mode. The ghosting was negligible.

Similar studies were performed by Bissonnette *et al.* [6]. They have shown that using the detector in a binned mode could allow a higher number of frames per second, increasing the total number of projections without increasing the examination time and obtaining images with less artifacts.

Recent developments

The future of breast tomosynthesis is still under discussion [7]. Many questions regarding the acquisition protocol are not completely addressed and other will arise in the future. For example, lowering slice thickness could increase the lesion detectability but, would simultaneously increase the number of images that the clinician would have to analyse. Some are trying to reduce this extra work for the clinicians by developing new Computer Aided Detection (CAD) algorithms especially designed for breast tomosynthesis. Until now, there were two kinds of solutions published: one that consists in detecting and scoring masses in reconstructed volumes [8, 9] and other that does the same directly from the tomosynthesis projections [10].

One of the developments to the tomosynthesis technique that is being tested is the use of contrast-enhancement techniques [11]. An initial clinical experiment has been published [12] in which a single bolus of iodinated contrast agent was administrated. With this, it was possible to obtain images of both morphologic and vascular characteristics of breast lesions comparable with the ones obtained by Magnetic Resonance Imaging.

In addition, some new applications will certainly be considered, such as tumour volume estimation or surgical planning with better depth localisation of lesions [7].

Image Reconstruction for Digital Breast Tomosynthesis (DBT)

The principle of tomosynthesis is the acquisition of multiple projections (2D) around the object, for different angles, providing, after image reconstruction, 3D information of that object. For that reason, tomosynthesis is a tomographic imaging modality.

The concept of conventional tomosynthesis was introduced by Ziedses des Plantes, in 1932, whose paper on geometric tomography is often considered as the introduction of tomographic imaging to the medical community.

In breast tomosynthesis, and contrary to computed tomography, projection images are acquired at a limited number of views over a limited angular range. The main reason for this incomplete sampling relies on the total dose, which, as was explained before, should be comparable to that used in conventional mammography. In consequence, the reconstruction of a 3D volume from the corresponding set of 2D projections is, in fact, a limited-angle cone-beam tomographic problem.

The first reconstruction algorithm adopted for tomosynthesis was the "*Shift-and-Add*" algorithm [1, 13]. From a computational point of view it is not a very demanding algorithm, and this was, by the time it appeared, a very important advantage. On the other hand, since its principles were already known from microscopy, the adaptation for tomosynthesis was rather straightforward.

The shift-and-add algorithm uses the fact that objects at different heights above the detector will experience different degrees of parallax as the X-ray tube moves, and, therefore, will be projected onto the detector at positions depending on the relative heights of the objects (Fig. 2). Based on this fact, knowing the geometrical relation between the object location on its original reconstruction plane and the corresponding position on each of the acquired projections, it is possible to shift and add images acquired during the tube movement such that structures in some plane are all made to become focused [13].

One should notice, however, the need of a logarithmic transform on projection data prior to reconstruction, in order to ensure that the linear combination of images in the shift-and-add method yields images with linear relationship to the objects in the plane of interest and the overlying anatomical blur [13]. Therefore, instead of using the value of I stored in each projection bin, reconstruction algorithms process $\ln(I)$.

In Fig. 2 we show how an object on the xz plane (normal to the rotation axis) is projected onto the detector, when the tube has an isocentric motion around the system's center of rotation and the detector is stationary. To calculate the amount of shift along the x axis that is necessary before adding and averaging, one needs to establish the equation with the geometrical relation between x and x_i, i.e., $x = x(z,x_i)$. Let L be the distance between the fulcrum and the x-ray-tube position and D the distance between the center of rotation and the image plane. Then, $tan(\theta) = \frac{Lsin\phi+x}{Lcos\phi+D-z}$, and, since $tan(\theta)$ can also be expressed as $tan(\theta) = \frac{x_i-x}{z}$, we get:

$$x_i = z.\left(\frac{Lsin\phi+x}{Lcos\phi+D-z}\right)+x \qquad \textbf{Eq. 1}$$

The shift of projections is based on Eq. 1 and the tomosynthesis image is the average of all *n* shifted projection images.

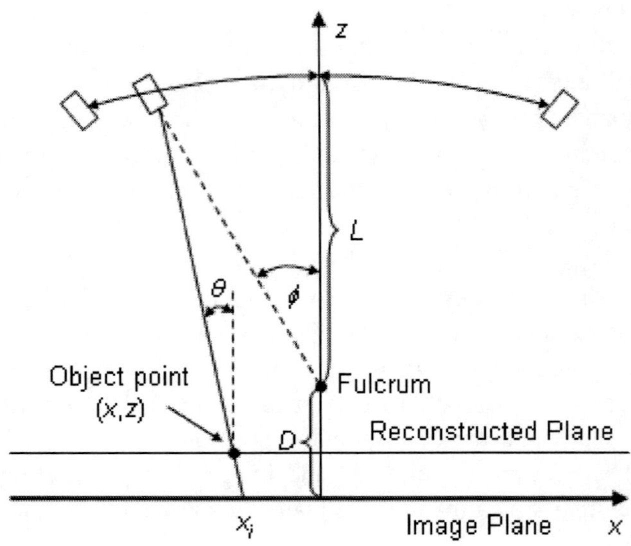

Figure 2. The geometry of the shift-and-add reconstruction for tomosynthesis.

One important drawback of the shift-and-add algorithm is the fact that reconstructed images contain not only objects of interest in the focal plane, but also blurred objects, from other planes, superimposed on the plane of interest. There are many methods described in the literature for reducing the blurred out-of-plane structures. Some of them are [13]: the spatial frequency filtering, ectomography, the selective plane removal, filtered back projection, matrix inversion tomosynthesis (MITS), and, even, iterative restoration methods (that should be not confused with true algebraic iterative image reconstruction algorithms).

The shift-and-add algorithm is an example of an analytical reconstruction algorithm. This means that after translating the reconstruction problem into a mathematical equation, the algorithm is designed in order to find the best analytical solution for that equation. Algebraic techniques are the alternative to analytical approaches. The distinctive feature of the latter type of algorithms is the fact that they iteratively refine the estimation of the attenuation coefficients. In addition, discretisation is not, as in the case of analytical methods, a contingence: data are assumed to be intrinsically discrete.

There are some issues that must be address when considering the use of an algebraic reconstruction algorithm. Fessler [14] clearly stated five requirements:

1. a finite parameterisation of the object, usually represented as a discrete set of voxels;
2. a model of the measurement, i.e., a system model, **l**, that relates the unknown coefficients to the expectation of each detector measurement;
3. a model of the measurement uncertainty, i.e., a model of the probability distribution of each measurement around its expectation value;
4. an objective function providing a measure of how well an image fits the data, that should be maximised (or, considering an alternative point of view, a distance to be minimised);
5. an iterative algorithm for maximising the objective function, including specification of the initial estimate and stopping criterion.

For each requirement, different choices have been adopted and, in consequence, different algorithms were devised.

The first step is the definition of a finite parameterisation of the object, resulting in a discrete set of voxels. Let the whole volume be subdivided into J voxels, and the linear attenuation coefficient for the jth voxel be denoted by u, $1 \leq j \leq J$. Considering a digital detector with I bins and assuming that number of rays is equal to the number of detector elements, the ith ray, $1 \leq i \leq I$, is defined as the line segment starting from x-ray source location to the center of the ith detector element. If, in addition, the path length of the ith ray going through the jth voxel in the nth x-ray tube location (projection view) is denoted by a_{ijn}, then it is possible to translate the projection/detection model into a matrix-vector equation:

$$\mathbf{l}_n . \mathbf{u} = \mathbf{y}_n \qquad \textbf{Eq. 2}$$

where: $\mathbf{l}_n$ is the projection matrix for the nth projection view with a_{ijn} as its (i,j)th element; and $\mathbf{y}_n$ is the corresponding vector of the projection data ($1 \leq n \leq N$, where N is the total number of projection views). This is the way to address the second requirement referred above, and Eq. 2 is the linear system model for the projection/backprojection core of algebraic techniques for image reconstruction.

For this particular subject, and since DBT is a transmission tomography technique, it should also be taken into consideration that the ith projection value, y_{in}, is proportional to the logarithmic transform of the ratio of the incident intensity ($I_{o,n}$) and the transmitted intensity ($I_{i,n}$) of the ith ray [15]:

$$y_{i,n} = k.\ln\frac{I_{0,n}}{I_{i,n}}$$ **Eq. 3**

The choice of a model for the measurement of uncertainty plays a fundamental role on the distinction between algebraic techniques. Even the absence of such a model is, by itself, a distinctive feature. In fact, if no model is assumed for the noise, an algebraic reconstruction technique can be classified as *non-statistical*, in opposition to *statistical iterative reconstruction (SIR) techniques*, a group including all the algebraic techniques incorporating any statistical model for the data. ART (Algebraic Reconstruction Technique) is an example of a non-statistical algorithm. Among SIR methods, differences rely on the statistical model adopted.

In ART, the linear attenuation coefficients are updated in a "ray-by-ray" manner, and all voxels along the ray under consideration are updated using the difference between the detected and computed bin value. This difference is backprojected along the ray and contributes to each voxel in proportion to the path length of the ray inside this voxel. Since the update is performed on a projection by projection basis, ART has fast convergence speed but the solution can be very noisy and is strongly affected by the ill-posed inverse problem, namely as a consequence of the limited-angle acquisition.

Variations of the original ART implementation have been devised, differing not only in the method used to update the current estimation, but also on the amount of information used to perform such update. In SART (Simultaneous Iterative Reconstruction Technique), the linear attenuation coefficient of each voxel will not be updated until after all rays in one projection view have been processed once and, therefore, the number of updates, after one complete iteration, is equal to the number of projection views *N*. In SIRT, the update is performed just after all projection views have been processed.

For iterative algebraic reconstruction techniques like SART, several aspects need to be considered. One of them is the initial values for the iterative process. Another is the selection of an appropriate step size or relaxation parameter. A third, and also of great importance, is the order through which projections are accessed. In fact, it has been suggested that the order of processed projections should be arranged such that successive projections are well "separated," i.e., having least correlation in term of information. For DBT, changing the access order of the projection views may not have strong effects on the reconstruction quality, since the number of projections is small and they are acquired over a limited angular range [15].

As stated before, the goal of algebraic reconstruction techniques is to iteratively find the best solution for the set of linear equations in Eq. 2, where "best" means the minimum error between measured and calculated projection data. While apparently simple, this is of great importance. Digging a little deeper on this subject, it becomes clear that, at first, it is necessary to clarify how the error is defined or, in other words, which is the distance that should be minimised in order to minimise the error. This is the role of the objective function. In fact, its expression can account for two different terms: one, that is always present for all statistical iterative reconstruction methods, gives a measure of how well the image fits the data; the other, controls how this image matches some desired properties (*a priori* constraints). Some authors [14] argue that objective functions based solely on the measurement statistics (Poisson or Gaussian) perform poorly due to the ill-conditioned nature of tomographic reconstruction. In particular, this sort of unregularised methods, i.e., methods whose objective function contains just the likelihood term, produce increasingly noisy images as the number of iteration also increases. So, these authors point the need for regularisation methods containing a term to impose a smoothness constraint on the reconstructed image. Explicit regularisation procedures include the introduction of a prior distribution through a Bayesian approach. If we designate this regularisation term by $R(\mathbf{u})$, then the general expression for the whole objective function could be as follows:

$$\Phi(\mathbf{y},\mathbf{u}) = L(\mathbf{y},\mathbf{u}) - \beta.R(\mathbf{u}) \qquad \textbf{Eq. 4}$$

where β is a parameter that controls the balance between the data fitting criterion and the image property criterion, that are not rarely conflicting goals [14].

If just the likelihood term is present, statistical iterative reconstruction methods are referred as non-Bayesian reconstruction methods. On the contrary, when the objective function in addition to the likelihood includes the regularised term, the reconstruction is said to be Bayesian. So, whenever a reconstruction method is said to be regularised, or penalised, it can also be classified as Bayesian.

The Maximum Likelihood – Expectation Maximisation is one example of a well known algebraic statistical, non-Bayesian, reconstruction algorithm. As the name suggests, the objective function to be maximised is the likelihood function, and the tool used to iteratively proceed towards the maximum likelihood is the expectation maximisation algorithm [16]. Vardi [17] discusses the relation between the maximum likelihood estimate and the minimum for the Kullback-Leibler information divergence function (assumed as a distance function), a relevant and appealing subject because it associates the maximum of the objective function with the minimum of a distance.

The likelihood function is the probability of getting the n measured projections, **y**, given a 3D model of attenuation coefficients **u**: $L = P(\mathbf{y}|\mathbf{u})$.

Assuming that the incident and transmitted x-rays follow a Poisson statistics, the likelihood function is given by:

$$L = \prod_i \{P_i(\boldsymbol{y}_i|\boldsymbol{u})\} = \prod_i \frac{e^{-\overline{y_i}}\overline{y_i}^{y_i}}{y_i!}$$

where: i is the detector bin; y_i is the value measured for bin i; and $P_i(\boldsymbol{y}_i|\boldsymbol{u})$ is the likelihood associated with each detector bin.

In order to use the former equation, one should first establish how to estimate $\overline{y_i}$, i.e., the number of photons expected at detector bin i, based on the attenuation model **u**. In other words, the mean number of photons in bin i. Considering the exponential attenuation of the x-ray beam along the path from source to detector, $\overline{y_i} = D_i e^{\langle l,u \rangle_i}$, where: D_i is the number of incident x-ray photons at bin i before attenuation; $\langle l,u \rangle_i = \sum_j l_{ij} u_j$ is the total attenuation along beam ray i; and l_{ij} is the intersection length of beam ray i and voxel j.

If the log-likelihood is used instead of the likelihood, then:

$$lnL = \sum_i \left(-D_i e^{-\langle l,u \rangle_i} - y_i \langle l,u \rangle_i + y_i lnD_i - ln(y_i!)\right)$$

The transmitted x-rays collected by the detector are ''incomplete information'' about the attenuation coefficient of image voxels along the beam ray. The expectation maximisation algorithm postulates a larger vector of unobserved complete data where the observed ''incomplete data'', **y**, is embedded. For a single projection data bin from the ''incomplete'' data space, this complete data space consists of the unobservable x-ray counts leaving each voxel along the beam ray from the source to the projection image bin [18]. Because ''complete data'' are not known, the EM algorithm uses their expectation based on the current estimate of the model.

There are two steps at each iteration of the EM algorithm: an expectation step (E-step) and a maximisation step (M-step). In the E-step, the ''complete data'' are estimated by calculating their expectation, given the ''incomplete data'' **y** and the current model **u**. In the M-step, the log-likelihood function of the ''complete data'' is maximised. These two steps can be resumed as follows [16, 19].

- E-step: estimation of the complete-data sufficient statistics, **x**, by means of the conditional expectation: $\hat{x}^{(p)} = E[\mathbf{x}|\mathbf{y}, \mathbf{u}^{(p)}]$;
- M-step: the former conditional expectation is maximised with respect to **u**, so $\mathbf{u}^{(p+1)}$ is determined as the solution of the equation: $E[\mathbf{x}|\mathbf{u}] = \hat{x}^{(p)}$

where $\mathbf{u}^{(p)}$ is a vector with the parameter's values after p iterations and $\hat{x}^{(p)}$ is one realisation of **x**.

The mathematical equations involved in both steps are intricate and beyond the scope of the present work. For those readers who are willing to take knowledge of the assumptions, mathematical reasoning and approximations behind the proposed iterative equation, we strongly recommend the papers by Lange and Carson [19] and Lange and Fessler [20]. Nevertheless, the core equation suggested by these authors is the following:

$$u_j^{(n+1)} = \frac{\sum_i (M_{ij} - N_{ij})}{1/2 \sum_i (M_{ij} - N_{ij}) l_{ij}} \qquad \textbf{Eq. 5}$$

where

$$M_{ij} = y_i + D_i \left[exp\left(-\sum_{k=1}^{j-1} l_{ik} u_k^{(n)}\right) - exp\left(-\sum_{k=1}^{k_{max}} l_{ik} u_k^{(n)}\right)\right]$$

is the expected number of photons entering pixel j and $N_{ij} = M_{i,j+1}$ is the expected number of photons leaving pixel j along the ray defined by projection bin i [21].

In spite of the alternative approaches (and corresponding assumptions) adopted to derive different versions of the iterative equation for the ML-EM reconstruction, for the sake of usefulness we believe it is important to mention those that were used specifically for DBT. That is the case of the implementation described by Wu [18], following one of the approaches suggested by Lange and Fessler:

$$u_j^{(n+1)} = u_j^{(n)} + \Delta u_j^{(n)} \qquad \textbf{Eq. 6}$$

where

$$\Delta u_j^{(n)} = \frac{u_j^{(n)} \sum_i l_{ij}\left(D_i e^{-\langle l, u^{(n)} \rangle_i} - y_i\right)}{\sum_i \left(l_{ij} \langle l, u^{(n)} \rangle_i D_i e^{-\langle l, u^{(n)} \rangle_i}\right)}. \qquad \textbf{Eq. 7}$$

The numerator of the voxel update, Δu_i, is proportional to the attenuation in the voxel. The update is, thus, multiplicative and a zero in any voxel should be avoided when initializing the model. The summed expression in the numerator represents the backprojection of the difference between the expected intensity, $D_i e^{-\langle l,u \rangle_i}$, and the observed intensity, y_i, in the projection images. This ''error term'' is backprojected into the voxel by multiplying by l_{ij} (the intersection of each projection ray with the voxel being updated). This error is also weighted by the factor in the denominator, which provides the minimum expected error under the assumption of Poisson noise in the observed projections.

Radiation Dose to Patients from Breast Tomosynthesis

The increased risks resulting from radiation dose after x-ray mammography have recently become of increased concern especially for genetically susceptible patients [22, 23]. It is therefore of particular importance to obtain detailed information about the factors that may be responsible for the radiation doses received by patients in tomosynthesis. In fact, since tomosynthesis obtains several planar projections of the breast to gain insight into the 3D anatomy, one could expect a sharp dose increase relative to planar mammography.

The radiation dose received by patients undergoing tomosynthesis is still a relatively unknown issue. In fact, only after some years of testing in a real clinical setting can we account for what may be different imaging procedures, essentially guided by medical doctors' experience and patient pathological conditions. Radiation doses in planar mammography have been studied thoroughly [24-34]. These studies showed, among other things, that for a single projection mammography, the mean glandular dose varies linearly with glandularity. However, these studies only take into account the craniocaudal view of the breast and, in tomosynthesis, one must consider acquisitions centred in the mediolateral oblique view. Furthermore, the variation of the glandular dose with the projection angle must be characterised. Sechopoulos et al [35] used Monte Carlo simulation methods in order to characterise the glandular dose during a tomosynthesis study. In this study, they took into account the possible variations in breast size, composition, x-ray spectrum and mammographic view. They have simulated the breast as a complex solid, which included a portion of the *pectoralis* muscle. The breast size was varied as it was varied the amount of glandular tissue constituting the breast. Sechopoulos et al were able to indicate that from their simulation data, the radiation dose to the breast tissue was conditioned by the amount of muscle being crossed by x-rays as well as for the fact that in oblique views, the breast seen by the x-ray tube is always bigger that in the craniocaudal view, which may result in an overall dose increase as compared to digital planar mammography. At about the same time, a group from the UK [36], used Monte Carlo simulation in order to estimate the mean glandular dose to the breast for a tomosynthesis system with different x-ray anode-filter combinations. They simulated 9 different breast sizes, 3 glandularities, 4 tube voltages and 15 projections. They also studied the effect of positioning the breast relative to the imaging detector in mediolateral oblique view. These authors showed that the total mean glandular dose resulting from tomosynthesis is approximately independent from the distance between the chest wall and the nipple. The mean glandular dose values obtained by this group was close to 5.2 mGy/mGy for a combination of W/Al+Ag filter, 30 kVp and a compressed breast thickness of 5 cm. Additionally, they concluded that from a dosimetric point of view, the mediolateral oblique view was better than the craniocaudal view. However, they also stated that there was the need to assess the problem in a real clinical setting as a function of detectability of lesions in the breast.

These studies catalysed the evaluation of variable dose tomosynthesis technique in which one half of the dose is used to acquire the central projection and the rest evenly distributed by the rest. The first group to propose this idea was the group of Nishikawa at the Chicago Medical Center [37] and Das *et al.* evaluated its performance using an imaging prototype and a mastectomy specimen [38]. This group devoted its attention to the problem of detecting ductal carcinoma *in situ* and in particular, to the issue of microcalcification detection, which is directly related to the ability of potentially contribute to the decrease of breast cancer mortality. The authors performed a study where they compared the use of a uniform dose tomosynthesis of 4 mGy distributed over 21 projections along a 30° arc and a 5 cm thick compressed breast, with the possible use of 2 mGy for a central projection while distributing the remaining 2 mGy by the other projections. This was additionally motivated from the fact that the tomosynthesis systems at test allow obtaining digital mammography and tomosynthesis data. In their work, these authors conclude that using a uniform dose approach is statistically better than using a variable dose technique while keeping the total mean glandular dose close to the value accepted to a two-view mammography examination (approximately 4 mGy for a 5 cm thick compressed breast). However this group states that the relationship among dose and microcalcification detection and the value of the dose at the central projection remains unclear since higher dose does not necessarily mean better detection and speculate that different dose distributions may be studied while keeping the total mean glandular dose constant.

More recently, Gang *et al.* [39], complemented the experimental results by producing a theoretical evaluation allowing optimising the detection in tomosynthesis and in cone-beam CT (which is also under research for applications to mammography [40-46]). They developed an analytical model observer based in simple imaging geometries and show that there are tradeoffs among anatomical background, quantum and electronic noise that need to be met in order to obtain the best quality data. This is, of course, dependent on the x-ray flux striking the patients, since this flux, especially for thick breasts, may determine lesion-to-background contrast and thus the radiation dose delivered to patients.

A Japanese group recently performed an evaluation of the effective radiation doses received while using a tomosynthesis system for chest imaging. This study was performed using thermoluminescent dosimeters inside an anthropomorphic phantom and reported doses inferior to 1 mSv for head, chest, abdomen and hip-joint scans. The use of tomosynthesis systems for other applications than mammography is still an open issue [47].

In spite of all this, and for practical acquisition purposes, the radiology community believes that due to the similarities between tomosynthesis and digital mammography, dosimetry in tomosynthesis can be seen as an "extension" of what happens in tomography, only with a small loss of accuracy.

Lesion detection is also influenced by image reconstruction [41, 48-51]. Iterative reconstruction algorithms, used in other imaging modalities requiring a limited number of data projections, are known to be able to model the detection process. This allows them to take into account the detection noise in a much more efficient way than analytical methods (e.g. filtered backprojection). The use of iterative algorithms in breast tomosynthesis may therefore be a useful tool to achieve noise reduction in the clinical setting while preserving lesion detection capabilities [15, 52-54].

Clinical Value of Digital Breast Tomosynthesis

In recent years, a few clinical studies have been done on the clinical value of Digital Breast Tomosynthesis. More comprehensive studies are needed in order to fully realise the clinical role of DBT and to accurately assess its added value to cancer detection and/or cancer diagnosis.

Poplack published in 2007 a clinical study performed with 98 women with the objective of comparing the image quality of the DBT with that of Digital Mammography (DM) [55]. For all women both CC and MLO views were acquired for DM and DBT was also acquired in the two views, CC and MLO and for one woman the two breasts were acquired. A total of 99 images were acquired. A Selenia equipment from Hologic (Massachusetts, USA) was used to produce 11 low-dose projection views within 11 seconds with an angular range of 28°. Images were interpreted by 6 clinical radiologists, which rated the equivalence (better, equal or worse) for a specific finding. Observers evaluated the images according to feature analysis specific to the finding type.

Results show that observers rated DBT images superior or equivalent to DM for various findings except for the case of microcalcifications. 13 out of 19 findings of breast masses in the DBT images were rated as superior to diagnostic mammography and 5 were rated as equivalent. As for architectural distortion 5 of the 7 cases found were rated as having equivalent quality in DBT and DM and the remaining 2 to have better quality in DBT. As for asymmetry, in 19 out of the 53 findings, the images were found to be superior to DM and in 33 of them deemed equivalent and only for one finding was judged that DBT quality was inferior to that of DM. In focal asymmetry one finding was registered as having better image quality in DBT and another one, out of 6, to have inferior image quality. Finally, for microcalcifications, just in 2 out of 14 cases DBT was considered to have better quality while in 4 cases was considered to have equivalent and in 8 to have inferior image quality when compared to diagnostic mammography. This seems to indicate that, globally (in 51 out of 99 cases) the image quality was considered equivalent in both techniques, but in 37 out of the 99 cases DBT image quality was considered superior and in 11 cases was considered inferior to diagnostic mammography. Additionally, when used as an adjunct of DM, DBT analysis resulted in a reduction of the recall rate, a reduction of 40% or 52% depending on the methodology used.

The authors concluded that, according to the radiologist's subjective judgment, DBT images were found to have an image quality equivalent or superior to that of DM in all kinds of findings but the microcalcifications. Although, authors stated that the length of the DBT acquisition and the thin reconstructed slices may have contributed to the poor performance for calcification characterisation. A short acquisition may contribute to minimise the chance of having motion-related blur and thicker slices may also play a role in a better evaluation of calcifications in DBT.

Andersson *et al.* published in 2008 a study where 40 cancers were imaged with DBT in 37 breasts of 36 women from a large screening population [56]. Women were selected upon suspicious findings based on screening Digital Mammography or Ultrasonography (US). Digital Breast Tomosynthesis was performed using only one view. The DBT view acquired was equal to the Digital Mammography view in which the finding was less visible. In the cases where the finding was only visible in ultrasound imaging, rather than DM, DBT was acquired in MLO view. DBT was performed in a prototype adapted from a Siemens Novation where the DM was acquired. The mean absorbed dose was 0.8 mGy for a single DM image and for DBT was twice that of the DM image. A total of 25 projection images were acquired in a 50 degrees angular range. Acquisition lasted 20 seconds per breast. Images were reviewed by two breast imaging radiologist experts to reach a reading consensus and all images were available in the same workstation. The suspicious findings were qualitatively rated as "not visible", "questionably visible", "visible" and "clearly visible".

Results show that, when compared to single-view DM, DBT was ranked higher in 22 of the 40 cancers. In 13 cancers both single-view DM and DBT were rated equally as "visible/clearly visible" and in just one case single-view DM was ranked higher than DBT. The 4 remaining cancers were not visible in both techniques. When compared with two-view DM, DBT was ranked higher in 11 cases, ranked equally, as "visible/clearly visible", in 24 cases and in just one case DM was better rated. The remaining 4 cases were visible neither in two-view DM nor in DBT.

The authors also compared BIRADS classification using the different techniques. As for single DM, DBT upgraded BIRADS classification in 21 patients: 11 of them from 1-2 to 3-5 and the remaining 10 from 3 to 4-5 in the BIRADS ranking. When compared with two-view DM, DBT resulted in an upgrade in 12 cases, 4 of them being upgraded from 1-2 to 3-5 and the other 8 being upgraded from BIRADS 3 to 4-5. The combination of two-view DM plus US was compared with DBT. It resulted in the changing of 2 cancers

BIRADS classification (upgraded) based on the use of DBT. In 7 other cases, the classification was downgraded with DBT. Four of these last 5 cases were only visible in the US examination.

The authors concluded that, whereas this was a non-blinded study, DBT provided a better visualisation of lesions and a more accurate BIRADS classification. In this study, when compared with two-view DM, Digital Breast Tomosynthesis increased tumour detectability.

On a different study [57], Smith *et al.* aimed to assess the clinical performance of DBT as a function of radiologist' experience. In this case, the comparison was made between DM and DM+DBT. There was no specific information on the conditions of the Digital Breast Tomosynthesis acquisition. Nevertheless, we acknowledge that for the main purpose of the study that information is not as relevant as it would be for a comparison of DM versus DBT.

The data was collected from 5 clinical centers and was composed by a selection of 316 images that included 48 cancers. The images were classified by 12 readers, all of them certified radiologists but with different experience levels. Experience was divided in three classes: "highly experienced", "experienced" and "less experienced". The performance of the readers was assessed with ROC curves for each scenario: DM and DM+DBT. The figure-of-merit Area Under the Curve (AUC) was used to quantitatively compare different curves. Additionally, the recall rates were also evaluated.

Results show that the AUC increases in all readers. The AUC measure increased from 0.823 to 0.901 in "highly experienced", from 0.838 to 0.878 in "experienced" and finally from 0.834 to 0.911 in the "less experienced" group. The plot of the amount increased as a function of the years since training and the amount of mammograms per year scrutinised showed no clear trend. As for the recall rate, a significant reduction was recorded: from 52.0% to 12.8% in "highly experienced", from 49.3% to 13.7% in "experienced" and from 52.3% to 12.6% in the "less experienced" group.

Authors concluded that DBT allows an increased performance when used as a complement to DM and that its usefulness can be seen for all radiologist's experience levels. It was found that all radiologists improve their performance with 3D by an amount that is independent from his or her experience.

In 2009, a study by Teertstra *et al.*, reported on the results of evaluating a total of 513 women with both mammography and tomosynthesis examinations [58]. According to the authors, the study intended to assess the potential value of tomosynthesis in women with an abnormal screening mammogram or clinical symptoms of breast cancer. The subjects were referred from a national screening program for a second opinion and accepted to participate in the study. Complementary ultrasound and biopsy were performed when needed.

A standard double-view examination was made for Digital Mammography with both CC and MLO views being acquired in a Lorad Selenia from Hologic. Tomosynthesis was also acquired in a Hologic prototype with a high-resolution detector comparable to that of DM. 11 images were collected from -7.5° do 7.5°. It is said by the authors that the total radiation exposure from DBT is comparable to a double-view DM examination.

The authors present their work as the first one to prospectively compare DBT sensitivity to that of Digital Mammography. Digital Breast Tomosynthesis detected 104 cancers and missed 8 cases lately confirmed as positives giving a sensitivity of 92.9%, the exact same result that it was registered for DM. And as for the negative cases, in DBT, 699 of them were correctly classified but there were 129 false positives resulting in a specificity of 84.4%, a little less than the 88.9% of DM, from 713 true negatives plus 115 false positives. The same results are shown as positive predictive value, 44.6% for DBT and 47.5% for DM and as negative predictive value, 98.9% for both DBT and DM.

The authors concluded that DBT can be used as a complement to DM since there were lesions detected in DBT that were missed by DM, but the authors stated that these lesions are also likely to be detected by other techniques. It is believed, after this study, that the clinical role of DBT is yet to be established.

Some ongoing clinical trial have already published some of the results[59-61]. Although, so far Good *et al.* concluded that DBT needs optimisation in order to clarify its clinical role [59], Gur *et al.* concluded that use of DBT may decrease the recall rate in a substantial amount [61] Finally, Hakim *et al.* concluded that DBT may be an alternative to obtain additional mammographic information e that in some cases may eliminate the need for ultrasound [60].

Recently, Gennaro *et al.* compared clinical performance of DBT in one view to the clinical performance of FFDM in the usual two views [62]. The 200 hundred women experiment was accomplished involving six breast radiologists with experience ranging from 5 to 30 years in breast imaging. The radiologists had a training period to become familiar with DBT images. After that period, the breasts radiologists evaluated the images from both DM and DBT in an anonymised and blinded test. Diagnostic accuracy of both techniques was assessed with area under the ROC curve figure of merit.

This study used a GE Senographe 2000 to make DM acquisition in CC and MLO views and a GE investigational prototype to make the single MLO

DBT acquisition. The prototype is based on the FFDM GE's equipment Senographe DS modified in order to acquire 15 projections between -20 and +20 degrees. More, it is said that that anode and filter, kVp and total mAs were defined as function of breast thickness so that the radiation dose for DBT in one view was equal to the radiation dose of the standard mammography in two views. Data was reconstructed using SART algorithm with 1 mm slices. Additional 10 mm slices were made available as a preview to the entire set.

Although 200 women participated in the trial only 376 breast were included due to technical problems during the acquisition or due to the presence of scars in the imaged breasts. It was found that 63 of them had malign lesions, 177 benign lesions and in 136 of them no lesion was present. A mean ROC curve was build from the 6 readers' analysis of the images. Values for AUC were obtained: 0.851 for DBT and 0.836 for FFDM. This difference was found not to be statistically significant.

As a conclusion, the authors stated that it was shown that, for the studied population, the techniques had similar clinical performances. Although it is said that non-inferiority statement is not sufficient to propose the replacement of FFDM by DBT, the authors consider the results encouraging although emphasising that DBT is not yet a mature technology. Finally, they also pointed out that review time may impair the usage of DBT in a screening environment.

List of Acronyms

AUC	Area Under the Curve
BIRADS	Breast Imaging-Reporting and Data System
CAD	Computer Aided Detection
CC	Craniocaudal
DBT	Digital Breast Tomosynthesis
DM	Digital Mammography
FFDM	Full-Field Digital Mammography
ML-EM	Maximum Likelihood – Expectation Maximisation
MLO	Mediolateral Oblique
ROC	Receiver Operating Characteristic
SART	Simultaneous Algebraic Reconstruction Technique
US	Ultrasonography

Clinical trials already done have no definite conclusions on DBT clinical value although it is clear it has a great potential to overcome some of the limitations pointed out to digital mammography and to improve cancer detection.

Bibliography

1. Niklason, L.T., et al., *Digital Tomosynthesis in breast imaging.* Radiology, 1997. **205**(2): p. 399-406.
2. Pisano, E.D. and M.J. Yaffe, *Digital mammography.* Radiology, 2005. **234**(2): p. 353-362.
3. Zhao, B. and W. Zhao, *Imaging performance of an amorphous selenium digital mammography detector in a breast tomosynthesis system.* Medical Physics, 2008. **35**(5): p. 1978-1987.
4. Sechopoulos, I. and C. Ghetti, *Optimization of the acquisition geometry in digital tomosynthesis of the breast.* Medical Physics, 2009. **36**(4): p. 1199-1207.
5. Zhao, B., et al., *Experimental validation of a three-dimensional linear system model for breast tomosynthesis.* Medical Physics, 2009. **36**(1): p. 240-251.
6. Bissonnette, M., et al., *Digital breast tomosynthesis using an amorphous selenium flat panel detector.* Medical Imaging 2005: Physics of Medical Imaging, 2005. **5745**: p. 529-540.
7. Park, J.M., et al., *Breast tomosynthesis: Present considerations and future applications.* Radiographics, 2007. **27**: p. S231-S240.
8. Chan, H.P., et al., *Computer-aided detection system for breast masses on digital tomosynthesis mammograms: Preliminary experience.* Radiology, 2006. **238**(1): p. 1075-1080.
9. Chan, H.P., et al., *Computer-aided detection of masses in digital tomosynthesis mammography: Comparison of three approaches.* Medical Physics, 2008. **35**(9): p. 4087-4095.
10. Reiser, I., et al., *Computerized mass detection for digital breast tomosynthesis directly from the projection images.* Medical Physics, 2006. **33**(2): p. 482-491.
11. Diekmann, F. and U. Bick, *Tomosynthesis and contrast-enhanced digital mammography: recent advances in digital mammography.* European Radiology, 2007. **17**(12): p. 3086-3092.

12. Chen, S.C., et al., *Initial clinical experience with contrast-enhanced digital breast tomosynthesis.* Academic Radiology, 2007. **14**(2): p. 229-238.
13. Dobbins, J.T. and D.J. Godfrey, *Digital x-ray tomosynthesis: current state of the art and clinical potential.* Physics in Medicine and Biology, 2003. **48**(19): p. R65-R106.
14. Fessler, J.A., *Penalized Weighted Least-Squares Image-Reconstruction for Positron Emission Tomography.* IEEE Transactions on Medical Imaging, 1994. **13**(2): p. 290-300.
15. Zhang, Y.H., et al., *A comparative study of limited-angle cone-beam reconstruction methods for breast tomosynthesis.* Medical Physics, 2006. **33**(10): p. 3781-3795.
16. Dempster, A.P., N.M. Laird, and D.B. Rubin, *Maximum Likelihood from Incomplete Data Via Em Algorithm.* Journal of the Royal Statistical Society Series B-Methodological, 1977. **39**(1): p. 1-38.
17. Vardi, Y. and D. Lee, *Discrete radon transform and its approximate inversion via the EM algorithm.* International Journal of Imaging Systems and Technology, 1998. **9**(2-3): p. 155-173.
18. Wu, T., et al., *Tomographic mammography using a limited number of low-dose cone-beam projection images.* Medical Physics, 2003. **30**(3): p. 365-380.
19. Lange, K. and R. Carson, *EM reconstruction algorithms for emission and transmission tomography.* Journal of Computer Assisted Tomography, 1984. **8**(2): p. 306-16.
20. Lange, K. and J.A. Fessler, *Globally Convergent Algorithms for Maximum a-Posteriori Transmission Tomography.* IEEE Transactions on Image Processing, 1995. **4**(10): p. 1430-1438.
21. Manglos, S.H., et al., *Transmission Maximum-Likelihood Reconstruction with Ordered Subsets for Cone-Beam Ct.* Physics in Medicine and Biology, 1995. **40**(7): p. 1225-1241.
22. Heyes, G.J., A.J. Mill, and M.W. Charles, *Mammography-oncogenecity at low doses.* Journal of Radiological Protection, 2009. **29**(2A): p. A123-A132.
23. Jansen-van der Weide, M.C., et al., *Exposure to low-dose radiation and the risk of breast cancer among women with a familial or genetic predisposition: a meta-analysis.* European Radiology, 2010. **20**(11): p. 2547-2556.

24. Kimme-Smith, C., et al., *New mammography screen/film combinations: imaging characteristics and radiation dose.* AJR Am J Roentgenol, 1990. **154**(4): p. 713-9.
25. Robinson, J.D., et al., *Improved mammography with a reduced radiation dose.* Radiology, 1993. **188**(3): p. 868-71.
26. Adcock, D.F. and D.B. Howe, *Radiation dose and risk in screening mammography.* J Med Syst, 1994. **18**(4): p. 173-8.
27. Thilander-Klang, A.C., et al., *Influence of anode-filter combinations on image quality and radiation dose in 965 women undergoing mammography.* Radiology, 1997. **203**(2): p. 348-54.
28. Haus, A.G. and M.J. Yaffe, *Screen-film and digital mammography. Image quality and radiation dose considerations.* Radiol Clin North Am, 2000. **38**(4): p. 871-98.
29. Pisano, E.D., et al., *Factors affecting increasing radiation dose for mammography in North Carolina from 1997 through 2001: an analysis of Food and Drug Administration annual surveys.* Acad Radiol, 2004. **11**(5): p. 536-43.
30. Ng, K.H., N. Jamal, and L. DeWerd, *Global quality control perspective for the physical and technical aspects of screen-film mammography--image quality and radiation dose.* Radiat Prot Dosimetry, 2006. **121**(4): p. 445-51.
31. Whitaker, C.J., et al., *Influence of menopausal status and use of hormone replacement therapy on radiation dose from mammography in routine breast screening.* Br J Radiol, 2006. **79**(943): p. 597-602.
32. Kuzmiak, C.M., et al., *Factors affecting decreasing radiation dose for mammography in North Carolina after 2002: an analysis of Food and Drug Administration annual surveys.* Acad Radiol, 2007. **14**(6): p. 685-91.
33. Samei, E., et al., *Digital mammography: effects of reduced radiation dose on diagnostic performance.* Radiology, 2007. **243**(2): p. 396-404.
34. Smathers, R.L., et al., *Radiation dose reduction for augmentation mammography.* AJR Am J Roentgenol, 2007. **188**(5): p. 1414-21.
35. Sechopoulos, I., et al., *Computation of the glandular radiation dose in digital tomosynthesis of the breast.* Med Phys, 2007. **34**(1): p. 221-32.
36. Ma, A.K., et al., *Mean glandular dose estimation using MCNPX for a digital breast tomosynthesis system with tungsten/aluminum and tungsten/aluminum+silver x-ray anode-filter combinations.* Med Phys, 2008. **35**(12): p. 5278-89.

37. Reiser, I., et al., *Development of a model for breast tomosynthesis image acquisition.* Medical Imaging 2007: Physics of Medical Imaging, Pts 1-3, 2007. **6510**: p. U1472-U1479.

38. Das, M., et al., *Evaluation of a variable dose acquisition technique for microcalcification and mass detection in digital breast tomosynthesis.* Medical Physics, 2009. **36**(6): p. 1976-1984.

39. Gang, G.J., et al., *Anatomical background and generalized detectability in tomosynthesis and cone-beam CT.* Med Phys, 2010. **37**(5): p. 1948-65.

40. Yang, D., R. Ning, and W. Cai, *Circle plus partial helical scan scheme for a flat panel detector-based cone beam breast X-ray CT.* Int J Biomed Imaging, 2009. **2009**: p. 637867.

41. Zhang, X., R. Ning, and D. Yang, *Cone Beam Breast CT noise reduction using 3D adaptive Gaussian filtering.* J Xray Sci Technol, 2009. **17**(4): p. 319-33.

42. Chen, L., et al., *Dual resolution cone beam breast CT: a feasibility study.* Med Phys, 2009. **36**(9): p. 4007-14.

43. Madhav, P., et al., *Evaluation of tilted cone-beam CT orbits in the development of a dedicated hybrid mammotomograph.* Physics in Medicine and Biology, 2009. **54**(12): p. 3659-3676.

44. Zeng, K., et al., *An in vitro evaluation of cone-beam breast CT methods.* J Xray Sci Technol, 2008. **16**(3): p. 171-187.

45. Karellas, A., J.Y. Lo, and C.G. Orton, *Point/Counterpoint. Cone beam x-ray CT will be superior to digital x-ray tomosynthesis in imaging the breast and delineating cancer.* Med Phys, 2008. **35**(2): p. 409-11.

46. Yang, K., A.L. Kwan, and J.M. Boone, *Computer modeling of the spatial resolution properties of a dedicated breast CT system.* Med Phys, 2007. **34**(6): p. 2059-69.

47. Koyama, S., et al., *Radiation dose evaluation in tomosynthesis and C-arm cone-beam CT examinations with an anthropomorphic phantom.* Medical Physics, 2010. **37**(8): p. 4298-4306.

48. Chen, B. and R. Ning, *Cone-beam volume CT breast imaging: feasibility study.* Med Phys, 2002. **29**(5): p. 755-70.

49. Lai, C.J., et al., *Visibility of microcalcification in cone beam breast CT: effects of X-ray tube voltage and radiation dose.* Med Phys, 2007. **34**(7): p. 2995-3004.

50. Sarkar, V., et al., *The effect of a limited number of projections and reconstruction algorithms on the image quality of megavoltage digital*

tomosynthesis. Journal of Applied Clinical Medical Physics, 2009. **10**(3): p. 155-172.

51. Wu, G., J. Mainprize, and M. Yaffe, *Characterization of projection ordering in iterative reconstruction methods for breast tomosynthesis.* Digital Mammography, Proceedings, 2008. **5116**: p. 601-605.
52. Wu, T., et al., *A comparison of reconstruction algorithms for breast tomosynthesis.* Medical Physics, 2004. **31**(9): p. 2636-2647.
53. Kastanis, I., et al., *3D digital breast tomosynthesis using total variation regularization.* Digital Mammography, Proceedings, 2008. **5116**: p. 621-627.
54. Reiser, I., B.A. Lau, and R.M. Nishikawa, *Effect of scan angle and reconstruction algorithm on model observer performance in tomosynthesis.* Digital Mammography, Proceedings, 2008. **5116**: p. 606-611.
55. Poplack, S.P., et al., *Digital breast tomosynthesis: Initial experience in 98 women with abnormal digital screening mammography.* American Journal of Roentgenology, 2007. **189**(3): p. 616-623.
56. Andersson, I., et al., *Breast tomosynthesis and digital mammography: a comparison of breast cancer visibility and BIRADS classification in a population of cancers with subtle mammographic findings.* European Radiology, 2008. **18**(12): p. 2817-2825.
57. Smith, A.P., E.A. Rafferty, and L. Niklason, *Clinical performance of breast tomosynthesis as a function of radiologist experience level.* Digital Mammography, Proceedings, 2008. **5116**: p. 61-66.
58. Teertstra, H.J., et al., *Breast tomosynthesis in clinical practice: initial results.* European Radiology, 2009.
59. Good, W.F., et al., *Digital breast tomosynthesis: A pilot observer study.* American Journal of Roentgenology, 2008. **190**(4): p. 865-869.
60. Hakim, C.M., et al., *Digital Breast Tomosynthesis in the Diagnostic Environment: A Subjective Side-by-Side Review.* Am. J. Roentgenol., 2010. **195**(2): p. W172-176.
61. Gur, D., et al., *Digital Breast Tomosynthesis: Observer Performance Study.* Am. J. Roentgenol., 2009. **193**(2): p. 586-591.
62. Gennaro, G., et al., *Digital breast tomosynthesis versus digital mammography: a clinical performance study.* European Radiology, 2010. **20**(7): p. 1545-1553.

In: Mammography:
Editors: A. Palmetti, R. Roux

ISBN 978-1-61470-589-5

Chapter 3

SOCIOECONOMIC AND HEALTHCARE SUPPLY STATISTICAL DETERMINANTS OF COMPLIANCE TO MAMMOGRAPHY SCREENING PROGRAMS: A MULTILEVEL ANALYSIS IN CALVADOS, FRANCE

Carole Pornet[1,2,3,3]***, Olivier Dejardin***[1,2,3]***,***
Fabrice Morlais[1,2,3]***, Véronique Bouvier***[1,2,3] ***and***
Guy Launoy[1,2,3]

[1] ERI 3 INSERM ''Cancers & Populations'', Faculty of Medicine, Avenue Côte de Nacre, 14032 Caen Cedex, France
[2] University of Caen EA3936, Department of Research & Evaluation in Epidemiology, Avenue Côte de Nacre, 14032 Caen Cedex, France
[3] CHU of Caen, Faculty of Medicine, Avenue Côte de Nacre, 14033 Caen Cedex, France

ABSTRACT

Background: Although the literature on factors associated with mammography screening is abundant, reasons for underparticipation

[3] E-mail address: carole.pornet@inserm.fr

remain unclear, most studies having focused exclusively on individual factors. This study aimed at investigating the ecological influence of socioeconomic status and healthcare supply on compliance to organized breast cancer screening programs, on an unbiased sample based on data from the entire target population within a French geographical area, Calvados (n = 98,822 women).

Methods: Individual data on participation and aggregate data on healthcare supply and socioeconomic status, respectively obtained from the structure responsible for organizing screening and the French census, were analyzed simultaneously using a multilevel model. Results: Uptake was lower among the youngest (50–54 years) and the oldest (70–74 years) women, compared to the intermediate 55–69 year age-group, with respectively OR = 0.73 (95%CI: 0.64–0.83) and OR = 0.78 (95%CI: 0.67–0.91). Uptake fell with increasing level of deprivation, a difference in uptake probability being observed between the least deprived and the most deprived areas (OR = 0.71; 95%CI: 0.59–0.86). Neither radiologist- nor primary care physicians-to-100,000 inhabitants ratios were associated with participation. Conclusions: Multilevel analysis allows to detect areas of weak participation statistically linked to areas of strong deprivation. So, even with organized breast cancer screening giving screening free of charge for target women, ecological socioeconomic factors have a more significant impact on participation than healthcare supply. These results suggest that targeting populations, in accurate geographical areas where women are less likely to participate, as identified socially and geographically in this study, could be adopted to reduce disparities in screening.

INTRODUCTION

Breast cancer is the main cause of mortality by cancer in women in France, responsible for 11,308 deaths in 2005 [1], and the second cause of mortality by cancer in women in the United Kingdom, responsible for 11,990 deaths in 2007 [2]. Randomized controlled trials have demonstrated that mammography screening reduces breast cancer mortality by 21% [3]. Similarly to many developed countries, except the United States [4,5], an organized breast cancer screening (BCS) program using mammography was set up in France in 1989, throughout 10 of the country's 96 geographical areas, referred to as ''departments'' [6]. This program was set up in 1996 in the Department of Calvados. In the French program, local screening management structures invited the target population, women aged from 50 to 74 years, by post to undergo a free mammography once every 2 years. Despite regular progress since the organized BCS program was generalized to include the entire French territory in 2004, the national rate of participation (52.5% in 2008) remains below European recommendations which advocate a 70% participation rate in order to obtain a significant reduction in mortality [6]. Although the literature on factors associated with mammography screening is abundant, the reasons for underparticipation remain unclear, most studies having focused exclusively on individual factors. The use of screening mammography has been described in previous conceptual models as being influenced by both individual and environmental characteristics [7–10]. Over the last decade, research has highlighted the influence of place of residence on behavior regarding screening, in particular BCS, and has increased awareness on the importance of considering ecological factors when studying individual behavior [7,8,10–17]. Whereas individual-level socioeconomic influence has been firmly established, influence of socioeconomic status (SES) of place of residence is conflicting across studies. Certain studies have reported that women in areas with higher SES [8,11,18,19], such as higher median incomes [13,20], higher rate of being gainfully employed [10] or higher school diplomas [20] demonstrated higher utilization rates. On the contrary, in other studies, no employment–population ratio influence was observed [7]. Findings regarding healthcare supply are also conflicting. Certain studies have reported that residing in a county with a greater number of physicians is associated with increased mammography [9,12], others observing no physician consultation rate influence [13,15]. To study influence of socioeconomic status of place of residence on behavior regarding screening with predictor variables measured simultaneously at different levels, multilevel analysis is pertinent. Indeed, taking into account the hierarchical structure of data, multilevel analysis allows to obtain more exact estimations of area-level variance than classical analysis. A number of North American and Swedish studies on ecological SES influencing screening mammography participation have used multilevel analysis [7,9,10,14,16,17,19]. Almost all of these studies were based on self-questionnaires on screening participation and were limited by participation bias; only the Swedish study was population-based [10]. However, this last study on uptake within an organized screening program did not take into account healthcare supply in its multilevel analysis. The aim of this study was to investigate if area-level SES and area-level healthcare supply were independent predictors of non-adherence to an organized mammography screening program within a representative sample of the target population, after controlling for individual characteristics using multilevel models.

MATERIALS AND METHODS

Study population

The study's target population, women aged from 50 to 74 years and resident within Calvados, included 98,822 subjects (Figure 1). Target population data were provided by the ''Association Mathilde'', in charge of organizing BCS in Calvados, a geographical area in Northwestern France. Data on identity and address had been initially provided to the association by the various health insurance organizations. The period of study was from 2004 to 2006. The availability of exact addresses enabled a geographical unit to be assigned to each participant (geocoding). The geographical units used were referred to as ''Ilo^ts Regroupe´ s pour l'Information Statistique'' (IRIS, or regrouped statistical information blocks), as defined by the National Institute for Statistics and Economic Studies (INSEE); they are the smallest geographical census units available in France.

Given that, in county-level models, a loss of significance had been highlighted for several contextual factors [17], the IRIS, the smallest-level model, was chosen. The regional capital and other major towns are divided into several IRISes and small towns form one IRIS. Our study zone, the Department of Calvados, counts a total of 829 IRISes (http://www.insee.fr).

Sampling of 5.5% of the target population was conducted, by simply drawing lots, without handing-over, and according to the law of uniform distribution. A total of 5375 women, for whom addresses were sufficiently complete, could then be geocoded (59 women had insufficiently complete addresses for geocoding) (Figure 1).

After geocoding, the final study population comprised 4940 women, 435 having been excluded, 299 of whom for medical reasons:

- Women with a normal mammography within the last year, without breast symptomatology (who were invited to perform a new mammography 22 months after the previous examination) and, consequently, likely to undergo an opportunistic mammography outside the screening program.

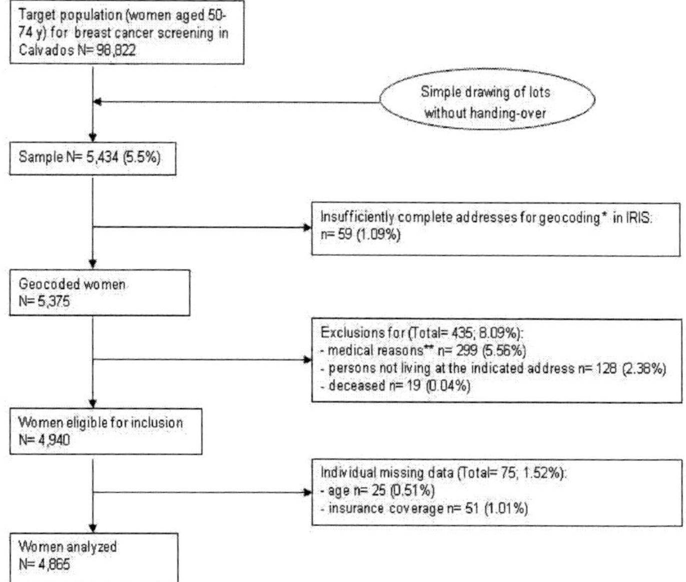

* Geocoding: attribution of a geographical unit for each subject thanks to the availability of exact address.
** Other care or screening strategies required for women at high-risk or very high-risk of breast cancer or for women having undergone opportunistic mammography within the last year.

Figure 1. Flow diagram.

- Temporary (i.e. medical supervision of a probably innocent abnormality) or permanently non-eligible women; in particular those benefiting from specific care during or after treatment for breast cancer, those benefiting from specific follow-up due to particular risk factors (carriers, or highly probable carriers of anoxious constitutional mutation predisposing to breast cancer), and women for whom a surgical act involving biopsy had evidenced a histological risk factor [21].

Final sample representativeness was checked in terms of participation rate, age and insurance coverage (Table 1).

Measurement methods

Participant or non-participant status was known for each woman (Table 2).

Table 1. Comparison between the final sample (n=4,940) and the target population (n=89,612[a])

	Final sample		Target population		Pearson χ^2
	n	%	n	%	
Participation in breast cancer screening					0.72; p>0.50
Yes	2,721	55.08	49,895	55.68	
No	2,219	44.92	39,717	44.32	
Age (years)					3.78; p>0.50
50-54	1,315	26.62	23,632	26.37	
55-59	1,184	23.97	21,817	24.35	
60-64	796	16.11	14,489	16.17	
65-69	777	15.73	13,849	15.45	
70-74	843	17.07	15,508	17.31	
Not known	25	0.51	317	0.35	
Insurance coverage [b]					8.58; p>0.10
CPAM	3,544	71.74	65,097	72.64	
Special coverage systems	100	2.02	1,685	1.88	
Civil servant systems	579	11.72	9,425	10.52	
Self-employed, independent occupations	300	6.07	5,586	6.23	
MSA	366	7.41	6,837	7.63	
Not known	51	1.03	982	1.10	

[a] The target population within Calvados for which mammography was effectively proposed was: 98,822 – 9,210 women having been excluded for medical reasons, for death or because they did not live at the indicated address.

[b] Different systems of insurance coverage exist in France: the most common is the general medical insurance scheme (CPAM), the "Mutuelle Sociale Agricole" (MSA) covering agricultural occupations, other coverage including civil servant systems. Special coverage systems concern individuals employed by major French organizations such as "Electricité de France" (EDF-French electricity board) and the "Société Nationale des Chemins de Fer" (SNCF-French railway company).

Table 2. Participation in breast screening and characteristics of the population study (n=4,865)

	Participation		No participation		P for Heterogeneity
	n	%	n	%	
Age (years)					<0.000 1
50-54	665	50.76	645	49.24	
55-59	688	58.55	487	41.45	
60-64	466	59.51	317	40.49	
65-69	443	57.68	325	42.32	
70-74	435	52.47	394	47.53	
Insurance coverage[a]					0.07
CPAM	1938	55.01	1585	44.99	
Special system	61	61.00	39	39.00	
Civil servant system	330	57.19	247	42.81	
Self-employed, independent occupations	150	50.00	150	50.00	
MSA	218	59.73	147	40.27	
Townsend index[b]					0.000 4
Quintile 1 (least deprived)	369	60.29	243	39.71	
Quintile 2	348	59.18	240	40.82	
Quintile 3	337	58.10	243	41.90	
Quintile 4	506	56.04	397	43.96	
Quintile 5 (most deprived)	1137	52.11	1045	47.89	
Radiologists / 100,000 inhabitants					0.14
=0	2446	55.78	1939	44.22	
>0	251	52.29	229	47.71	
PCP / 100,000 inhabitants					0.51
=0	1029	56.05	807	43.95	
>0	1668	55.07	1361	44.93	

[a]Different systems of insurance coverage exist in France: the most common is the general medical insurance scheme (CPAM), the "Mutuelle Sociale Agricole" (MSA) covering agricultural occupations, other coverage including civil servant systems. Special coverage systems concern individuals employed by major French organizations such as "Electricité de France" (EDF-French electricity board) and the "Société Nationale des Chemins de Fer" (SNCF-French railway company). [b]Quintiles of the Townsend index were calculated from the distribution of IRISes within the Calvados area as such quintile 5 represented 20% of the most deprived IRISes, but 45% of the population study.

Participants were defined as having undergone screening mammography within the duration of the study.

Two types of variables were used, individual and aggregate.

Level-1 individual variables: age and insurance coverage were obtained from exhaustive registries held by the ''Association Mathilde'' and via all health insurance organizations within Calvados (Table 2). In France, medical insurance coverage is virtually universal. Homeless women were excluded from our population study (as well as women living in mobile homes) due to lack of address which was crucial for sending the screening invitation. Unemployed and retired women were included in our population study, since they had an available address. Different systems of insurance coverage exist in France: the most common is the general medical insurance scheme (CPAM), the ''Mutuelle Sociale Agricole'' (MSA) covering agricultural occupations, other coverage including civil servant systems, schemes for the self-employed or other specific systems. Special coverage systems concern individuals employed by major French organizations such as ''Electricite´ de France'' (EDF—French electricity board) and the ''Sociéte´ Nationale des Chemins de Fer'' (SNCF—French railway company).

Level-2 aggregate variables: each woman was assigned the socioeconomic characteristics for her appropriate neighborhood (IRIS-level) using French census data provided by the INSEE in 1999. The INSEE produces a large number of socioeconomic indicators. Consequently, since deprivation is multifactorial [22], the selection of relevant variables for the determination of the SES of each IRIS proved difficult. Therefore, a composite index of deprivation, less sensitive to measurement bias than individual variables considered independently, was used [23]. The Townsend index, [22], which is widely used and acknowledged in Anglo-Saxon countries, was chosen [23]. This index is based on the unweighted sum of four centred and reduced socioeconomic variables, after log-transformation of the first 3: percentage of overcrowned households, percentage of households without a car, percentage of unemployed individuals of an economically active age, and the square root of the percentage of non-home owner households. To allow international comparisons, a standardized division into quintiles of the distribution of the Townsend index score for each IRIS was carried out: quintile 1 representing the most privileged IRIS and, conversely, quintile 5, the most deprived. Each woman was assigned the radiologist-to-100,000 inhabitants ratio and primary care physician (PCP)-to-100,000 inhabitants ratio for her appropriate neighborhood (IRIS-level). Healthcare supply was estimated by radiologist- and PCP-to-100,000 inhabitants ratios with in numerator: the number of radiologists (PCP) and in denominator: 100,000 inhabitants for each IRIS [24]. Radiologists practicing in public or private centres were approved to perform screening mammographies. Since the distribution of the radiologist- and PCP-to-100,000 inhabitants for each IRIS was highly asymmetric, these two ratio variables were dichotomised by their geometric means.

Statistical analysis

The influence of aggregate data and individual data on screening mammography compliance, dependent variable (participation vs. non-participation), was analyzed, firstly using univariate logistic regression, then two-level (multilevel) logistic regression models with individuals (level-1) residing within the IRISes (level-2). The adopted modeling strategy consisted in increasing model complexity at each step, using a random intercept model [25]. All statistical analyses were performed using the SAS system, the NLMIXED procedure being used for multilevel models (Statistical Analysis System software, version 9.1, Cary, NC, USA).

Since, within organized systems, it had been highlighted that women participating in opportunistic screening had a higher educational level than those participating in organized screening [26,27], we compared the SES of the area of residence for the 4940 women comprising our study population to that of the 299 women excluded for medical reasons, among them, women with a normal mammography within the last year, without breast symptomatology, and likely to undergo an opportunistic mammography.

Finally, the demographic characteristics of the 128 women not living at the indicated address were compared to those of the women included in the study using Chi-squared tests.

RESULTS

Among the 4865 women studied, 55.4% participated in organized screening mammography during the period 2004–2006. BCS participation and population study characteristics are summarized in both Table 2 and the univariate model in Table 3. Uptake was significantly lower in the youngest (50–54 years) and in the oldest (70–74 years) age-groups, in comparison to the intermediate (55–69 years) age-group, with respectively OR = 0.73 (95%CI: 0.64–0.83) and OR = 0.78 (95%CI: 0.67–0.91). The distribution of health insurance coverage was close significant between participants and non-participants ($p = 0.07$). In the univariate model in Table 3, participants more frequently benefited from CPAM coverage, special coverage, significantly civil servant systems or MSA than from self-employed and independent occupation coverage systems. Among level-2 variables, only the Townsend index had a significant statistical influence on participation ($p < 0.0001$); neither radiologist- nor PCP-to-100,000 inhabitants ratios being significantly associated with participation (respectively, $p = 0.14$ and $p = 0.36$). The variables successively added in multilevel models were those significantly linked with participation at a threshold of 0.10, i.e., age, insurance coverage and Townsend index. BCS participation varied significantly according to IRIS (test of random intercept: $p = 0.01$) (Table 3, empty model). Adjustment for level-1 variables slightly decreased differences between IRISes by 1.5%, signifying that disparities in inter-IRIS participation could barely be explained by these individual factors (Table 3, model 1). Addition of the Townsend index to the model (Table 3, model 2) reduced the inter-IRIS variance by 47.3%, signifying that SES explained approximately half of the disparities between IRISes. Participation in least deprived IRISes (IRISes belonging to the quintile 1 of Townsend index; reference category) was higher than in most deprived IRISes [IRISes belonging to the quintile 5 of Townsend index; OR = 0.71 (95%CI: 0.59–0.86)]. Quintiles 2–4 of the Townsend index, representing the ''average'' socioeconomic category, had a negative statistical influence on participation compared to the first quintile, however, this association was borderline and with no marked linear decreasing trend from one quintile to another. On the contrary, a sharply significant negative association was observed between the 5th quintile of the Townsend index representing the most deprived socioeconomic category and participation. No statistically significant interaction between individual and aggregated variables was observed.

The SES of area of residence for the 4940 women comprising our study population was compared to that of the area of residence for the 299 women excluded for medical reasons. The latter resided as often within the most privileged IRISes (9.7%) and the most deprived IRISes (44.2%) as the study population (respectively 12.5% and 44.8%; $p = 0.50$), hence offering no information on the impact of area of residence on the likelihood of undergoing opportunistic mammography. We also compared the demographic characteristics of the 128 women not living at the indicated address to those of our study population. Women not living at the indicated address were no different from the study population with regard to mean age (respectively, 61.4 years vs. 60.6 years) and age distribution into 5 groups ($df = 4$; $x2 = 2.68$; $p =$

0.61), however their insurance coverage was more often unknown (26.56% vs. 1.03%, $p < 0.0001$).

DISCUSSION

The current study, based on a representative sample from a target population, adds to the relatively sparse but expanding literature on the role of ecological factors in organized BCS, by evaluating, at an accurate level, the factors related to socioeconomic influence and to the availability of PCPs and radiologists approved to perform screening mammographies. These results confirm the positive statistical relationship between low SES of place of residence and low rates of screening mammography, whereas healthcare supply was not statistically associated with participation in organized screening mammography programs.

This study presents some relevant methodological advantages. The use of area-based socioeconomic measurements allowed the enhancement of cancer screening management structure data, hence enabling the inclusion of additional indicators that are not routinely captured in screening management structure systems. Moreover, the use of aggregated socioeconomic data protects the study from the unavoidable selection bias observed in studies using self-questionnaires. Since many of the socioeconomic variables identified in the majority of studies as being associated with decreased mammography, such as income and education, are probably collinear, it is consequently difficult to determine the extent to which they are due to SES vs. individual factors [28]. The use of a composite deprivation index, such as the Townsend index, would appear to be more appropriate than independently considered variables in estimating socioeconomic influence on participation. Furthermore, the use of data on participation or nonparticipation obtained from a screening organization provided us with information on actual attitudes, hence protecting analysis from the risk of measurement bias, which is more common when using self-questionnaires [29]. Finally, our randomly composed sample is representative of the population concerned by organized BCS.

Several study limitations should, however, be noted. The quality of lists of eligible participants within organized systems varies from one country to another. Contrary to population registers, considered as the ideal source of eligible participants and used within organized programs in Nordic European countries [10], French national health insurance lists are neither up-to-date nor adequately representative of certain ethnic minority groups, and are often inaccurate, particularly in inner city areas, where population mobility is high. Consequently, the only putative bias regarding the representativeness of our sample derives from persons not living at the indicated address. The latter did not differ from those included in our study in terms of age. Nevertheless, persons not living at the indicated address are likely to be more mobile than those included in our study, and consequently not enjoying the strong social network that may positively influence health-related behavior. As such, their inclusion would have reinforced our conclusions. A limitation shared by many studies on neighborhood effects is the use of administrative census data as a proxy for neighborhood. It is unlikely that census boundaries directly coincide with any meaningful definition of ‘‘neighborhood’’ as defined by residents. However, there are several advantages in using census data, such as the systematic collection of data for the entire population and its accessibility. Moreover, our method for determining healthcare supply, via radiologist- or PCP-to-100,000 inhabitants ratios, fails to account for possible incongruence between IRIS of residence and IRIS of medical service provider or facility, since medical service provider catchment areas do not necessarily correspond to IRIS boundaries. We measured healthcare supply based on the number of radiologists approved to perform screening mammographies and available within the IRIS of residence, thus assuming that screening mammographies are performed within the same IRIS. In this study, we used a deprivation index, referring to a population and not to individuals. Consequently, a classification bias of individuals within IRISes can be suspected. Such bias could not be controlled in our analysis. A few rare area-based measurements (n = 18 IRISes), either SES or radiologist- and PCP-to-100,000 inhabitants ratios, were available at town-level, but not at IRISlevel, due to the lack of correspondence between these 18 IRISes and address. Use of town-level data to estimate area-level measurements almost certainly resulted in reduced accuracy [17]. However, this concerns only 2.2% of cases, and, consequently, has a very low decisive influence on results. IRIS-specific social characteristics applied to eligible women in 2004–2006, were drawn from the last exhaustive French census dating from 1999; potential changes in such characteristics over the study period could, therefore, not be taken into account. Finally, a limitation of this study based on the lack of person-level socioeconomic variables preventing from differentiating the effects of aggregated SES from person-level SES. So, we are not in position to conclude if the relationship between area and screening rate of participation is due to that rich people tend to live in certain areas (compositional effect).

Table 3. Socioeconomic factors of participation in breast cancer screening campaigns within a French geographical area, Calvados (2004-2006) – Multilevel Analysis (n= 4,865)

	Univariate model			Empty mo	Model 1			Model 2		
	OR[a]	95%CI[c]	p°		OR[a]	95%CI[c]	p°	OR[a]	95%CI[c]	p°
Fixed effects										
Level-1: individuals										
Age (years)			<.0001				<.0001			<.0001
50-54	1				1			1		
55-59	1.37	1.17-1.61			1.36	1.16-1.60		1.37	1.17-1.61	
60-64	1.43	1.19-1.71			1.45	1.21-1.74		1.46	1.22-1.75	
65-69	1.32	1.10-1.58			1.31	1.09-1.58		1.35	1.12-1.62	
70-74	1.07	0.90-1.27			1.07	0.89-1.28		1.10	0.92-1.31	
Insurance coverage			0.07				0.07			0.12
CPAM	1				1			1		
Special system	1.28	0.85-1.92			1.28	0.84-1.93		1.30	0.86-1.96	
Civil servant system	1.09	0.91-1.30			1.07	0.89-1.28		1.06	0.88-1.26	
Self-employed, independent occupations	0.82	0.65-1.03			0.80	0.63-1.02		0.80	0.63-1.01	
MSA	1.21	0.97-1.51			1.20	0.96-1.50		1.14	0.90-1.42	
Level-2: IRISes										
Townsend index			<.0001							<.0001

Table 3. Continued

Quintile 1 (least deprived)	1					1
Quintile 2	0.95	0.76-1.20				0.94
Quintile 3	0.91	0.72-1.15				0.90
Quintile 4	0.84	0.68-1.03				0.82
Quintile 5 (most deprived)	0.72	0.60-0.86				0.71
Radiologist/population			0.14			
=0/100,000 inhabitants	1					
>0/100,000 inhabitants	0.87	0.72-1.05				
PCP/population			0.36			
=0/100,000 inhabitants	1					
>0/100,000 inhabitants	0.95	0.84-1.07				
Random effects						
Level-2 variance (SD*)	-			0.0532 (0.028)	0.0524 (0.029)	0.0276 (0.02
D1 (D0)**	-			6681.4 (6686.7)	6641.5 (6652.2)	6624.3 (6631.9)
LRS χ^2 (p)[†]	-			5.29 (0.01(	10.74 (0.0005)	7.64 (0.002ξ
PCV[‡]	-			-	1.50%	47.33%

[a] OR: odds ratio [b] ORa: adjusted odds ratio [c] CI: confidence interval ○ P-trend: probability for categorial variables; P- heterogeneity: probability for non-ordering variables

*SD: standard deviation **D1: deviance of multilevel model with random intercept; D0: deviance of logistic model without random effect. † LRS: test of random intercept=D0-D1. Under the H_0, the statistics of LRS follows a distribution of χ^2 in 1df with p-value=0.5 of that indicated in the table of distribution of χ^2 in 1df. ‡ PCV: proportional change in variance at different levels=[(V1-V2)/V1]*100, where V1 is the level-2 variance of the multilevel model M1 with m1 variables and V2 the level-2 variance of the adjusted multilevel model M2 with m2=m1+1 variables.

Nevertheless, even if the reason for such association (rich people tend to live in certain areas or effect of ''environment'' even after taking into account individual and ecological socioeconomic position) is clearly unknown in this study, this study allows us to detect geographical units with a low rate of screening uptake. The identification of such area is the first step in the way to propose public health intervention for increasing screening uptake in all these area.

Contrary to the United States, where there is no national BCS program [14,16], in this French study, socioeconomic factors strongly statistically influenced mammography utilization and tended to be even more important than physician supply, as in Australia, Canada and the UK, other countries with established national BCS programs [11,13,18]. The magnitude of the statistical association between the Townsend score and screening mammography participation in our study was similar to that estimated in the only other study using the Townsend index, conducted in the UK, with an OR of 0.64 (95%CI: 0.59–0.70) in the most deprived compared to the least deprived category, and also with a significant test for trend ($p < 0.0001$) [18].

In our study, healthcare supply, represented by radiologist- and PCP-to-100,000 inhabitants ratios, measuring availability, was not statistically associated with participation; contrary to a US multilevel study, where the number of PCPs per 10,000 residents remained independently associated with screening mammography after accounting for aggregated and individual socioeconomic characteristics [9]. This absence of relationship is in keeping with a recent American multilevel analysis [17] and a geographical Canadian analysis [13], respectively using primary care provider shortage areas and numbers of mammography facilities per 1000 elderly women.

Conclusion

The methodology described here has the ability of applying modeling techniques to prospectively identify communities with the potential of becoming areas of low adherence with regard to BCS. Ultimately, this information could be used to develop effective interventions aimed at reducing disparities by assisting patients in cancer continuum, such as the North American patient navigator model in which the patient navigator are persons selected from the community who are trained to guide patients to receive appropriate services throughout the healthcare system [30].

ACKNOWLEDGMENTS

Calvados census data were provided thanks to the ''Centre Maurice Halbwachs'' (www.cmh.ens.fr). We also thank the ''Association Mathilde'' for having provided their data set.

REFERENCES

[1] French center of epidemiology on the medical causes of death (CépiDC). Interrogations des données (1979–2006) – Données détaillées – Available from: http://www.cepidc.vesinet.inserm.fr [accessed on 03 September 2010].

[2] Cancer Research UK. CancerStats key facts on breast cancer. Available from:http://info.cancerresearchuk.org/cancerstats/types/breast/#mortality [accessed on 03 September 2010].

[3] Nyström L, Andersson I, Bjurstam N, Frisell J, Nordenskjöld B, Rutqvist LE. Long-term effects of mammography screening: updated overview of the Swedish randomised trials. Lancet 2002;359:909–19.

[4] Hendrick RE, Klabunde C, Grivegne A, Pou G, Ballard-Barbash R. Technical quality control practives in mammography screening programs in 22 countries. Int J Qual Health Care 2002;14:219–26.

[5] Miles A, Cockburn J, Smith RA, Wardle J. A perspective from countries using organized screening programs. Cancer 2004;101(Suppl. 5):1201–13.

[6] French National Institute for Public Health Surveillance (Institut de Veille Sanitaire). Evaluation épidémiologique du programme de dépistage du cancer du sein. Available from: http://www.invs.sante.fr/surveillance [accessed on 03 September 2010].

[7] Kothari AR, Birch S. Individual and regional determinants of mammography uptake. Can J Public Health 2004;95:290–4.

[8] Dailey AB, Kasl SV, Holford TR, Calvocoressi L, Jones BA. Neighborhood-level socioeconomic predictors of nonadherence to mammography screening guidelines. Cancer Epidemiol Biomark Prev 2007;16:2293–303.

[9] Litaker D, Tomolo A. Association of contextual factors and breast cancer screening: finding new targets to promote early detection. J Women's Health 2007;16:36–45.

[10] Zackrisson S, Lindström M, Moghaddassi M, Andersson I, Janzon L. Social predictors of non-attendance in an urban mammographic screening programme: a multilevel analysis. Scand J Public Health 2007;35:548–54.

[11] Hyndman JCG, Holman CDJ, Dawes VP. Effect of distance and social disadvantage on the response to invitations to attend mammography screening. J Med Screen 2000;7:141–5.

[12] Benjamins MR, Kirby JB, Bond Huie SA. County characteristics and racial and ethnic disparities in the use of preventive services. Prev Med 2004;39:704–12.

[13] Glazier RH, Creatore MI, Gozdiyra P, Matheson FI, Steele LS, Boyle E, et al. Geographic methods for understanding and responding to disparities in mammography use in Toronto, Canada. J Gen Intern Med 2004;19:952–61.

[14] Rosenberg L, wise LA, Palmer JR, Horton NJ, Adams-Campbell LL. A multilevel study of socioeconomic predictors of regular mammography use among African-American women. Cancer Epidemiol Biomark Prev 2005;14:2628–33.

[15] Coughlin SS, Leadbetter S, Richards T, Sabatino SA. Contextual analysis of breast and cervical cancer screening and factors associated with health care access among United States women, 2002. Soc Sci Med 2008;66:260–75.

[16] Lian M, Jeffe DB, Schootman M. Racial and geographic differences in mammography screening in St. Louis City: a multilevel study. J Urban Health 2008;85:677–92.

[17] Mobley LR, Kuo TM, Andrews L. How sensitive are multilevel regression findings to defined area of context? A case study of mammography use in California. Med Care Res Rev 2008;65:315–37.

[18] Maheswaran R, Pearson T, Jordan H, Black D. Socioeconomic deprivation, travel distance, location of service, and uptake of breast cancer screening in North Derbyshire, UK. J Epidemiol Community Health 2006;60:208–12.

[19] Schootman M, Jeffe DB, Baker EA, Walker MS. Effect of area poverty rate on cancer screening across US communities. J Epidemiol Community Health 2006;60:202–7.

[20] Engelman KK, Hawley DB, Gazaway R, Mosier MC, Ahluwalia JS, Ellerbeck F. Impact of geographic barriers on the utilization of mammograms by older rural women. J Am Geriatr Soc 2002;50:62–8.

[21] French National Institute for Public Health Surveillance (Institut de Veille Sanitaire). Cahier des charges relatif à l'organisation du dépistage des cancers, aux structures de gestion, aux radiologues, annexes à la convention-type entre les organismes d'assurance maladie et les professionnels de santé′. Bull Off 2001.43. Available from: http://www.invs.sante.fr/surveillance [accessed on 03 September 2010].

[22] Townsend P. Deprivation. J Soc Policy 1987;16:125–378.

[23] Krieger N, Williams D, Moss N. Measuring social class in US public health research: concepts, methodologies and guidelines. Annu Rev Public Health 1997;18:341–78.

[24] Guagliardo MF. Spatial accessibility of primary care: concepts, methods and challenges. Int J Health Geogr 2004;3:3. Available from: http://www.ij-healthgeographics.com/content/3/1/3 [accessed on 03 September 2010].

[25] Pornet C, Dejardin O, Morlais F, Bouvier V, Launoy G. Socioeconomic determinants for compliance to colorectal cancer screening. A multilevel analysis. J Epidemiol Community Health 2010. published online 8 Sep 2009; doi:10.1136/jech.2008.081117.

[26] Duport N, Ancelle-Park R, Boussac-Zarebska M, Uhry Z, Bloch J. Are breast cancer screening practices associated with sociodemographic status and healthcare access? Analysis of a French cross-sectional study. Eur J Cancer Prev 2008;17:218–24.

[27] Esteva M, Ripoll J, Leiva A, Sanchez-Contador C, Collado F. Determinants of non attendance to mammography program in a region with high voluntary health insurance coverage. BMC Public Health 2008;8:387. doi: 10.1186/1471-2458/8/387.

[28] Schueler KM, Chu PW, Smith-Bindman R. Factors associated with mammography utilization: a systematic quantitative review of literature. J Women's Heath 2008;17:1477–98.

[29] Cronin KA, Miglioretti DL, Krapcho M, Yu B, Geller BM, Carney PA, et al. Bias associated with self-report of prior screening mammography. Cancer Epidemiol Biomark Prev 2009;18:1699–705.

[30] Wells KJ, Battaglia TA, Dudley DJ, Garcia R, Greened A, Calhoun E, et al. The Patient Navigation Research Program Patient naviagation: state of the art or is it science? Cancer 2008;113:1999–2010.

In: Mammography:
Editors: A. Palmetti, R. Roux
ISBN 978-1-61470-589-5

Chapter 4

MAMMOGRAPHY RESEARCH IN THAILAND

Viroj Wiwanitkit
Wiwanitkit House, Bangkhae, Bangkok, Thailand

ABSTRACT

Mammography is a useful tool for searching of breast abnormality. This investigation plays important role in reduction of rate of breast malignancy in many countries. In Thailand, mammography is also available for years and there are some interesting researches and reports on mammography in Thailand. However, those local publications are limited accessed by international society. Here, the author summarizes and discusses on some important researches on mammography in Thailand. This work can be useful data for further referencing in oncology.

INTRODUCTION

There are many applications of classical X ray techniques in the present day. Some applications are developed in order to serve specific purpose. A technique called "mammography" is an application in this category. Mammography is a useful tool for searching of breast abnormality [1 – 5]. This is a kind of X ray study focusing on the breast, a specific organ of human body. The detection of abnormal calcification within breast tissue is an important principle concept of mammography [1 – 5]. At present, this investigation plays important role in reduction of rate of breast malignancy in many countries. Although there are many reports on some limitations of the mammography, this tool is still accepted for its clinical usefulness [1 – 5]. It is an actual hope to fight breast cancer.

In Thailand, mammography is also available for years [6]. This tool is available in many large hospitals serving the requirement of local physicians [6]. It is expected that this tool is the new hope to control of breast cancer in Thailand [6]. There are some interesting researches and reports on mammography in Thailand. The data from those local reports are interesting and reflect geographical specific characteristics, a tropical developing country. However, those local publications are limited accessed by international society. Here, the author summarizes and discusses on some important researches on mammography in Thailand. This work can be useful data for further referencing in oncology and laboratory medicine.

REPORTS ON TOOL

A basic kind of reports on mammography is on the characteristic of the investigative tool, the X-ray mammogram. Indeed, this tool has a basic concept based on the classical X-ray tool but specially designed for specific purpose of breast examination. The important Thai reports are presented in Table 1.

Table 1. Some important reports on X ray mammogram tool in Thailand

Authors	Details
Thai Department of Medical Service [6]	This is an introductory paper on the X ray mammogram tool for the general readers, the local physician who work in different kinds of local hospitals in Thailand [6]. This is an early piece of publication on mammography in Thailand [6].

It should be noted that there are only a few reports on this aspect in Thailand. The question is “why there are only a few reports?” Indeed, this might be a common nature of developing countries that have limitation on technology development. Many developing countries including to Thailand have to "buy" technology from the developed countries. Buying means directly import technology without development in the country. No chance that new technique can be created if the technology is completely imported. Hence, it is not surprising that there is no report on development of mammography technology in Thailand. The reason might be the already mentioned reason. The existed reports are usually on the description of the technology, which can be called as "introductory" paper on new technique. The aim is to make the readers recognize on the new technology and correctly use it in the future. When the mammography technology reached Thailand, an introductory paper was also written and published by Thai Department of Medical Service [6]. This paper [6] is further used as a referencing paper on this topic for Thailand.

REPORTS ON DIAGNOSTIC PROPERTY

A basic group of student on any new diagnostic tool is on its diagnostic properties. This should describe on sensitivity, specificity, accuracy and predictive value. Indeed, this kind of report in important in laboratory medicine. Since the diagnostic property can be determined by several factors such as studied sample size, setting and environmental factors. The reports on diagnostic property from different settings are useful for help readers to judge on the exact usefulness of the tool.

Of interest, there are more papers on diagnostic property of mammography than those on "tool". This can restate the nature of developing country of Thailand. Indeed, developing countries usually study and publish paper on diagnostic property of the newly imported tools into their countries. This kind of papers still has advantages. Since it cannot completely expect on the actual diagnostic property of the newly developed tools on its first implementation, the continuous assessment and evaluation of the tool from several settings is required. The data can fulfill the missed or incomplete information on the diagnostic property of the tool. In Thailand, several reports can confirm the acceptable diagnostic property of the mammography. This can imply that the tropical geography pattern does not seriously affect the diagnostic property of the mammography. In addition, some Thai researches also reported on the combination of the mammography with the ultrasonography [8 – 9]. Improved diagnostic property could be seen based on this combination [8 – 9].

Table 2. Some important reports on diagnostic property of mammography in Thailand

Authors	Details
Fuangtharnthip et al. [7]	Fuangtharnthip et al. reported on subtle finding analysis in false negative results on screening mammogram based on their experience in a tertiary hospital in Thailand [7]. This report can reflect the considerable high rate of false positive and lead to the awareness on using of mammography [7].
Teavirat et al. [8]	Teavirat et al. reported on the diagnostic performance of combined mammogram and ultrasound in diagnosis of breast cancer [8]. Teavirat et al. concluded that this combination led to an improvement on diagnostic property [8].
Fuangtharnthip et al. [9]	Fuangtharnthip et al. reported on interval cancer in mammogram screening incidence and diagnostic value of additional ultrasonography in Thai women [9]. Similar to the report by Teavirat et al, Fuangtharnthip et al. concluded that the combination led to an improvement on diagnostic property [9]. This report is not only a paper on diagnostic property of mammography but also a paper on clinical application of mammography [9].

However, an interesting point that can be observed is on the lack for the cost effectiveness evaluation on the mammography. Indeed, cost effectiveness analysis is an important step in assessment of diagnostic property of the new tool. This approach can help judge on the appropriateness to invest on the new diagnostic tool. This kind of research is usually lacked in the developing countries. Although the developing countries usually have limited resource, they usually forget to perform this important step on evaluation of new diagnostic tools. How to promote the concept on complete evaluation of the new diagnostic tool for the developing settings is the topic to be discussed. How to make the local physicians or medical scientists in the developing countries to recognize on the need to adequately invest on the newly imported diagnostic tool is also another topic to be concerned.

REPORTS ON CLINICAL APPLICATION

This might be the most important group of researches. This kind of research reports the exact clinical application of the mammogram in clinical practice. The report on clinical application covers wide range of study. This includes epidemiology and clinical correlation of the findings from the investigation. This kind of research is an actual medical study. It is recommended that any new investigation has to be evaluated and assessed on clinical application. Without the data, it cannot judge that the newly developed investigation is clinically useful.

There are some reports on clinical applications of mammography in Thailand. Both studies on epidemiology and clinical correlation of the findings from mammographic test can be seen. The nature of the researches is usually a report from a single institute with a few subjects. This might decrease the generalization of the data from the reports. The big obstacles might be due to the lack of expertise in the research methodology and limited resource to perform the clinical research in Thailand. However, the reports in this area are still further useful for both local and international implications.

Table 3. Some important reports on clinical application of mammography in Thailand

Authors	Details
Fuangtharnthip et al [9]	Fuangtharnthip et al. reported on interval cancer in mammogram screening incidence [9]. This is a paper describing the epidemiology of breast cancer based on mammography [9]. Also, this paper described on the diagnostic property of mammography [9].
Boonjunwetwat and Prathombutr [10]	Boonjunwetwat and Prathombutr reported on mammographic findings of benign papillary neoplasm of the breast [10]. According to this work, mass and dense breast are the two common mammographic findings [10].

Table 3. Continued

Authors	Details
Tipsunthornsak [11]	Tipsunthornsak reported on the relatonship between microcalcification on mammogram and abnormal echogenic mass from ultrasound in the diagnosis of invasive ductal carcinoma [11].
Daungkaew [12]	A significant correlation was reported in this published paper [12]. Daungkaew reported on clinical experience on using mammogram in a local Thai provincial hospital namely "Saraburi Hospital" [12]. Daungkaew concluded that mammogram was actually useful in clinical practice in this setting [12]. This paper is a good example of the report from a non university tertiary hospital in Thailand. Although the author of this report is not an academic personnel in university, the author can still perform a good clinical study on mammography.
Muttarak et al. [13]	Muttarak et al. reported on role of mammography in diagnosis of axillary abnormalities in women with normal breast examination [13]. This is an interesting report on diagnosis of extra-breast lesion [13].
Ponstha et al. [14]	Ponstha et al. reported on mammographic changes related to different types of hormonal therapies [14]. Different patterns can be seen in different types of hormonal therapies [14].

CONCLUSION

Although mammography has been introduced to Thailand for years, the reports on mammography in Thailand are still limited. There are several reasons for this finding. There are some interesting reports on mammography in Thailand. Most are on the diagnostic property and clinical application. The lack of researched on the "tool" can be seen. It is recommended that further researches are required to fulfill the knowledge on mammography in Thailand.

REFERENCES

[1] Berlin L, Hall FM. More mammography Radiology. 2010 May;255(2):311-6.
[2] Nattinger AB. In the clinic. Breast cancer Ann Intern Med. 2010 Apr 6;152(7):ITC41.
[3] Hooks MA. Breast cancer South Med J. 2010 Apr;103(4):333-8.
[4] Balu-Maestro C, Chapellier C, Souci J, Caramella T, Marcotte-Bloch C. Breast cancer. J Gynecol Obstet Biol Reprod (Paris). 2010 Feb;39(1):3-10
[5] Gøtzsche PC, Nielsen M. Screening for breast cancer Cochrane Database Syst Rev. 2009 Oct 7;(4):CD001877.
[6] Mammogram. Bull Dept Med Serv. 1998 May ; 23(5): 265-266.
[7] Fuangtharnthip P, Viravan N, Bhothisuwan W, Augsusinha T. Subtle finding analysis in false negative results on screening mammogram and US : An institute study. Siriraj Med J. 2005 Aug; 57(8): 319-323.
[8] Fuangtharnthip P, Viravan N, Bhothisuwan W, Hargrove N, Nuchnapang Marikatat N, Augsusinha T. Interval cancer in mammogram screening incidence and diagnostic value of additional ultrasonography in Thai women. Siriraj Med J. 2005 Jul; 57(7): 257-261.
[9] Teavirat S, Hirunvivathanakul V, Jedsadapatharakul S. Diagnostic performance of combined mammogram and ultrasound in diagnosis of breast cancer. Vajira Med J. 2002 May; 46(2): 115-123.
[10]Boonjunwetwat D, Prathombutr A. Imaging of benign J Med Assoc Thai. 2000 Aug;83(8):832-8.
[11]Tipsunthornsak S. The relatonship between microcalcification on mammogram and abnormal echogenic mass from ultrasound in the diagnosis of invasive ductal carcinoma. Khon Kaen Hosp Med J. 2008 Jan-Apr; 32(1): 63-70.
[12]Daungkaew W. Mammogram in Saraburi Hospital. Saraburi Hosp Med J. 2003 Sep-Dec; 28(3): 124-133.
[13]Muttarak M, Chaiwun B, Peh WC. Role of mammography in diagnosis of axillary abnormalities in women with normal breast examination. Australas Radiol. 2004 Sep; 48(3): 306 – 10.

[14]Pongsatha S, Muttarak M, Chaovisitseree S, Luewan W, Panpanit A. Mammographic changes related to different types of hormonal therapies. J Med Assoc Thai. 2006 Feb; 89(2): 123 – 9.

In: Mammography:
Editors: A. Palmetti, R. Roux

ISBN 978-1-61470-589-5

Chapter 5

THE ROLE OF MAMMOGRAPHY IN THE PRE- AND POSTOPERATIVE REDUCTION MAMMOPLASTY PATIENT: A REVIEW OF THE LITERATURE

Jennifer R. Stevane, Michael J. Campbell and Keith T. Paige
Virginia Mason Medical Center, Seattle, Washington, U. S.

INTRODUCTION

Of all plastic surgery procedures, reduction mammoplasty has one of the highest satisfaction rates. Over 200,000 women of all ages undergo this procedure each year in the United States. The Surveillance Epidemiology and End Results (SEER) database estimated that in 2009, 190,000 women would be diagnosed with breast cancer, and over 40,000 women would die of the disease . Screening mammography can detect asymptomatic early stage breast cancer, but despite the popularity of breast reduction surgery and the commonness of breast cancer, there is no standardized, accepted means of using mammography for evaluating reduction mammoplasty patients before surgery, or following these patients long-term for screening and diagnostic purposes. This lack of guidance has led to an assortment of different approaches by surgeons in their use of mammography in this patient population.

This chapter will discuss the current research on these issues and give suggestions to the practioners who perform reduction mammoplasties for improved surveillance and management of these patients.

Preoperative Surveillance

During reduction mammoplasty, significant volumes of breast tissue are excised for success of the operation. Since reduction mammoplasty usually results in significant rearrangement of the parenchymal architecture, breast-sparing options are limited or impossible when adenocarcinoma of the breast is incidentally found in the reduction specimen. Therefore, detecting breast cancer prior to undergoing breast reduction remains of paramount importance.

Overall incidence of occult breast cancer in reduction mammoplasty specimens is less than 1% on average. Higher rates are noted when both invasive carcinomas and noninvasive pathologies such as ductal carcinoma in situ are included. Dotto and colleagues evaluated pathological slides from 516 bilateral reduction mammoplasties over a 15 year period. They found that the more concerning pathologies are found in patients over 40 years old, in women with a personal or family history of breast carcinoma, or in women with other predisposing factors [1].

In a retrospective review by Caldwell and colleagues, those women undergoing reduction mammoplasty with a personal history of breast cancer surgery on the other breast had reduction specimens with carcinoma 1.2% of the time. Alternatively, patients having a reduction for macromastia had only 0.7% positive specimens [2].

Precancerous and risk lesions can also be found in reduction mammoplasty specimens. Clark et al who reviewed over 500 reduction specimens found atypical ductal and lobular hyperplasias were in 4.4% of all patients, LCIS in 0.7%, and DCIS in 1.1%. There was no significant difference found in the incidence between benign and atypical histologies in those with and without a personal history of breast cancer. This did not hold true, however, for in situ carcinomas, where those with a past history of breast cancer had a statistically higher incidence [3].

The role of screening mammography prior to reduction mammoplasty remains subject to debate. The American Cancer Society guidelines state every woman should have a dedicated breast physical exam every 3 years starting in her twenties, followed by yearly mammograms stating at age forty [4]. Women with greater than normal risk should discuss the role of earlier imaging surveillance and MRI as an adjunct study with their physicians. Currently, there is no guidance as to the role of screening mammography prior to reduction mammoplasty. Generally, family and personal risk factors derived from the patient's history and the physical exam drive the decision to pursue preoperative screening mammography. Additionally, those due for a mammogram per nationally recognized screening recommendations should undergo this prior to surgery. Unfortunately, there is limited research on this topic. Gottlieb et al argued for a preoperative mammogram in addition to a thorough history and physical exam. They concluded that preoperative diagnosis would have avoided difficult intraoperative decisions regarding proceeding with reduction versus abandoning the operation, inadvertent tumor cell spillage, or affecting possible oncologic reconstruction from the reduction done [5].

Considering the pros and cons of preoperative mammography, what are practicing surgeons doing for their patients in the preoperative setting? In a study out of the Netherlands, a survey showed that up to 10% of surgeons did not physically palpate the breast for abnormalities prior to surgery, and many who did often did so in the setting of a positive personal or family history for breast cancer. Few surgeons required preoperative mammogram of all patients. Conclusions from that study advocated standard preoperative screening mammography for all patients 40 years or older to match screening recommendations for all women [6]. Similar conclusions have been suggested by others as the ideal means of preoperative surveillance and added that those who have significant personal or family risk factors should be imaged regardless of age [7].

Campbell and colleagues recently published a retrospective study on the influence of preoperative mammography in women considering breast reduction. Two hundred and seven women who underwent preoperative screening mammography prior to breast reduction surgery were evaluated over a five-year period. Thirty-two (16%) patients were found to have abnormal preoperative mammography, all of which were categorized as false positives. Abnormal imaging did not significantly influence the decision to proceed with reduction mammoplasty, but did have a trend toward delaying surgery. Similarly, preoperative mammography had no significant association with breast pathology discovered at time of reduction mammoplasty. The study concluded that preoperative mammography prior to reduction mammoplasty can detect the rare occurrence of breast cancer, but will also result in a high number of patients with false positive mammography. Surgeons should council their patients before obtaining preoperative mammography as to the high incidence of false positive studies and the need for subsequent diagnostic imaging[8].

Thus, it is suggested that patients considering reduction mammoplasty adhere to the standard guidelines for breast cancer surveillance. For patients under 40 years old it is imperative for the surgeon to conduct an interview to elucidate these risks followed by a physical exam to determine the need for a preoperative screening mammogram. If the patient is over 40 years old, the patient should have a recent screening mammogram as per American Cancer Society screening guidelines and the surgeon should council the patient as to the relatively high rate of false positives in the macromastia patient population. Even if surgery is delayed for further work-up, the patient will have been adequately evaluated and every attempt made to avoid an intra-operative diagnosis of cancer or a missed diagnosis that would have required different therapeutic approach.

Postoperative Surveillance

Post-reduction changes are well acknowledged and taken into account when radiologists study mammograms of patients having undergone this surgery. Multiple studies have helped to establish the expected postoperative changes seen on mammography and contributed to radiologists' ability to delineate those alterations from that caused by a malignant process. General categories include soft tissue change- retraction, skin changes, distortions and asymmetry, irregular margins, abnormal lucencies; and calcifications- found in areas of maximal operative trauma [9]. Calcifications seem to present slightly later than the soft tissue changes and, in contrast with malignant calcifications, are isolated, round, scattered, not clustered, and in areas of greatest parenchymal trauma. Keeping this and the patient's postoperative course in mind, when is the ideal time to initiate breast imaging and evaluate the changes, creating a baseline to future comparisons? A study from 1995 followed postoperative changes for up to 30 months and found that the calcification burden did not increase over the extended period of time, supporting a waiting period of at least 6 months prior to a postoperative mammogram which is the our current practice [10]. Brown, et al suggested postoperative mammography at 3 and 6 months to evaluate postoperative change [11]. This conclusion was supported by Beer and colleagues, who suggested 3 months as a sufficient time lapse to establish an adequate baseline mammogram [12]. More recently, Danikas et al [13] published a patient series evaluating the parenchymal changes seen on postoperative mammography in 118 patients. These images demonstrate that changes are apparent at 6 months with permanent features at 18 months surveillance. These include minimal breast tissue deep to the nipple-aerolar complex, shifting of the gland to a dependent position and an appearance of nipple elevation, parenchymal scarring and calcifications in areas of hematoma and suture lines, and fat necrosis emulating areas of suspicious findings such as cystic structure with rim calcifications. It is imperative to correlate the type of reduction mammoplasty technique with any abnormal findings to account for postoperative change versus concerning pathology. It is suggested, based on these findings, that a breast reduction patient undergo mammography at 6 months after surgery to image the acute postoperative changes, with another mammogram at 18 months to establish baseline comparison films after the postoperative scarring has formalized and is permanent.

Despite the numerous radiographic changes of reduction mammoplasty, there does not seem to be a difference in the sensitivity of mammography between those having had this operation and those who have not. In a recent case control study by Roberts et al, evaluation of 87 women who underwent reduction mammoplasty found that despite the substantial tissue mobilization performed during reduction mammoplasty, screening mammography in the first year following this operation does not lead to significantly more imaging or diagnostic interventions when compared with non-operative controls. In a larger retrospective review of over 200,000 breast reduction patients who had screening postoperative mammograms done in Australia, Muir and colleagues found no difference in recall rates between the surgical and non-surgical groups. Furthermore, of those who were diagnosed with malignancy via these mammograms, there was no significant difference between the types or location of the tumors [14]. Our group is currently working on a study in which reduction mammoplasty patients followed for a mean of five years have similar recall rates to those of nonoperative controls (unpublished data). There are times, of course, when the mammographic findings are equivocal. It is suggested that the physician proceed down the usual algorithm with diagnostic mammography, ultrasound, and biopsy. The postoperative nature of the breast should not preclude such investigations.

There is a need to establish a postoperative baseline mammogram for future comparisons although clearly there is no overall consensus as to the timeline of the needed imaging. Additionally, these women need to follow the appropriate guidelines for their age based on the American Cancer Society recommendations. The practice at our institution is a first postoperative mammogram between 6 and 12 months after reduction mammoplasty and then as per routine American Cancer Society guidelines.

Discussion

At a minimum, patients considering reduction mammoplasty should have a thorough history taken to elicit pertinent past personal and family histories and a comprehensive breast exam. If the patient has any significant history suggestive of a breast malignancy, regardless of *age,* preoperative mammography should be considered. Regardless of *history*, guidelines set forth by the American Cancer Society, for breast cancer screening should be followed. In addition to a discussion about the need for mammography, a discussion about the influence of the surgery on overall cancer risk should be mentioned. The incidence of breast cancer declines with removal of breast tissue, and the protective effect is most pronounced if the reduction mammoplasty is done after the age of 50 [15]. The amount of breast tissue removed correlates with the change in risk [16]. Lund, Ewertz, and Schou demonstrated that the greatest risk reduction occurred after 10 years surveillance when the volume of tissue removed was greater than 600g bilaterally [17].

Optimal timing of postoperative mammography is still debated. Postoperative changes are usually predictable and overall postoperative mammogram recall rates appear to be similar to those of women who do not undergo surgery. However, obtaining a baseline screening mammogram in the 3-12 months following breast reduction is probably warranted and may serve as a valuable comparison study in the future for these patients.

Screening mammography remains a vital tool in the preoperative evaluation and postoperative surveillance of the reduction mammoplasty and its role will continue to be defined in this growing patient population.

REFERENCES

[1] Dotto J et al. Frequency of clinically occult intraepithelial and invasive neoplasia in reduction mammoplasty specimens: A study of 516 cases. Int J Surg Pathol 16(1): 25-30, 2008
[2] Colwell AS et al. Occult breast carcinoma in reduction mammaplasty specimens: 14-year experience. Plast Reconstr Surg 113: 1984, 2004
[3] Clark CJ et al. Incidence of precancerous lesions in breast reduction tissue: A pathologic review of 562 consecutive patients. Plast Reconstr Surg 124:1033, 2009
[4] American Cancer Society Guidelines
[5] Gottlieb et al. Occult breast carcinoma in patients undergoing reduction mammaplasty. Aesth Plast Surg 13:279-283, 1989
[6] Hage JJ, Karim RB. Risk of breast cancer among reduction mammaplasty patients and the strategies used by plastic surgeons to detect such cancer. Plast Reconstr Surg 117: 727, 2006
[7] Clugston PA et al. Detecting breast cancer after reduction mammoplasty. CJS 34(1) Feb 1991
[8] Campbell MJ et al. The role of preoperative mammography in women considering reduction mammoplasty: a single institution review of 207 patients. Am J Surg 199(5): 636-640, 2010
[9] Clugston PA et al. Detecting breast cancer after reduction mammoplasty. Can J Surg 1991 Feb;34(1):37-40
[10]Abboud M et al. Incidence of calcifications in the breast after surgical reduction and liposuction. Plast Reconstr Surg 96(3):620-626, Sept 1995
[11]Brown FE et al. Mammographic changes following reduction mammoplasty. Plast Reconstr Surg 1987 Nov;80(5):691-8
[12]Beer GM et al. Diagnosis of breast tumors after breast reduction. Aesth Plast Surg 1996;20:391-397
[13]Danikas D et al. Mammographic findings following reduction mammaplasty. Aesth Plast Surg 2001;25:283-285
[14](Muir TM et al. Screening for breast cancer post-reduction mammoplasty. Clin Radiol. 2010 Mar;65(3):198-205
[15]Boice JD et al. Breast cancer following breast reduction surgery in Sweden. Plast Reconstr Surg 2000 Sept;106(4):755-762
[16]Brinton et al. Breast cancer risk in relation to amount of tissue removed during breast reduction operations in Sweden. Cancer 2001;91(3):478-483

[17]Lund K et al. Breast cancer incidence subsequent to surgical reduction of the female breast. Scand J Plast Reconstr Surg Hand Surg. 1987;21(2):209-12

In: Mammography:
Editors: A. Palmetti, R. Roux
ISBN 978-1-61470-589-5

Chapter 6

AN INTEGRATED APPROACH TO DESIGNATE THE SHORTAGE AREAS FOR MAMMOGRAPHY ACCESS IN A GIS ENVIRONMENT

Dajun Dai
Department of Geosciences, Georgia State University, Atlanta, GA, U. S.

ABSTRACT

Routine access to screening mammography is critical to detect the early malignancies and to reduce breast cancer mortality. This research aims to develop an approach to define areas short of mammography access by integrating both spatial and nonspatial factors in a Geographic Information Systems (GIS) environment. First, the spatial accessibility is measured on the basis of a Gaussian-based two step floating catchment area method. Second, the nonspatial accessibility is assessed by consolidating a variety of socioeconomic variables collected from Census 2000 into three factors (socioeconomic disadvantages, high social status, and high screening needs) using factor analysis. Finally, spatial access and nonspatial access are integrated into a designation scheme to define areas with poor access to mammography screening services. This approach may help public health professionals designate shortage areas to access mammography facilities, identify the factors responsible for poor access, and develop programs based on available resources.

Keywords: mammography access; shortage designation; Geographic Information Systems; spatial analysis; two-step floating catchment area method; factor analysis

INTRODUCTION

Breast cancer is a major public health problem and the second leading cause of cancer death in the United States. In 2009, it is estimated that more than 254,000 women were diagnosed with breast cancer and more than 40,000 women died from this disease (American Cancer Society, 2009), including approximate 192,370 new invasive cases (i.e., late-stage cases) and 62,280 cases of in situ breast cancer (i.e., early stage cases). The use of mammography has been effective for detecting the early malignancies and has significantly reduced breast cancer mortality (Breen et al., 2007; Elkin et al., 2010). Previous studies indicated that each year 4,475 deaths from breast cancer could be prevented if all eligible Americans received cancer screening services (Baron et al., 2008; Institute of Medicine, 2003). The prevalence of mammography among women with ages equal to or older than 40 years, however, has declined in recent years and caused the concern for increased cancer mortality (Barton, 2001; Breen et al., 2007).

Disparities in access to mammography have been a particular concern in the U.S. According to the U.S. Department of Health and Human Services (DHHS), the goal of Health People 2010 was to reach a 70% screening rate for all eligible women (DHHS, 2000). Yet the screening rates vary in different regions and among different ethnic and socioeconomic groups (Cronan et al., 2008; Jackson et al., 2009). Mammography access may be classified as revealed access and potential access (Luo & Wang, 2003). The former deals with the actual use of the screening services and the later sheds light on the probability (or opportunity) that one may use a service. This research focuses on the potential access because opportunities available to a woman have direct influences on the actual utilization of the offered services. Potential mammography access includes both spatial access and nonspatial access. Spatial access emphasizes the geographic barriers. Long-time traveling, for instance, may discourage women to routinely seek mammography screening services. Nonspatial access is related to demographic, socioeconomic, and ethnic factors (e.g., age, income, and race). Previous studies (Elkin et al., 2010; Wells & Roetzheim, 2007) suggested that age, education, income, health insurance, among others, were consistently related to screening mammography. The strong interactions between spatial and nonspatial access are persistent. Residents in close proximity to mammography facilities might be constrained by low incomes and could not afford screening services. In contrast, women from high-income families might not mind to drive a few miles to seek a preferred screening service. It would be critical to consider both spatial and nonspatial factors as well as their interactions when defining areas short of mammography screening services.

Many efforts have been made to delineate shortage areas of primary care physicians, but little has been done to designate shortage areas of mammography screening services. DHHS defines Health Professional Shortage Areas (HPSAs) as having shortages of primary care, dental or mental health providers. For example, it uses a population to practitioner ratio of 2,000:1 as the primary care HPSAs. For details, see guidelines at http://bhpr.hrsa.gov/shortage/ (last accessed 3 November 2010). Researchers (Luo & Wang, 2003; Wang & Luo, 2005) argued that the population to practitioner ratio is a regional availability measure which assumes the residential boundaries are impermeable. In other words, it assumes residents in one region (e.g., a county) will only use the health care services within this region. Yet people in reality may use health care resources in a neighboring region (e.g., a neighboring county) especially if they live near the border of the two regions. To address this issue, Luo and Wang (2003) proposed a two-step floating catchment area approach (2SFCA) which has been commonly used in health-care accessibility studies (Cervigni, Suzuki, Ishii, & Hata, 2008; Guagliardo, 2004; Langford & Higgs, 2006). The 2SFCA assumes equal access within a catchment, thus leading to the advancement—the Gaussian 2SFCA—in a recent study (Dai, 2010). The Gaussian 2SFCA applies a travel friction to discount the accessibility using a Gaussian function within each catchment. The advanced approach is effective to identify the areas short of spatial access to primary care physicians and mammography facilities. Wang and Luo (2005) integrated spatial and nonspatial factors to examine accessibility to primary care. They used the 2SFCA to measure spatial accessibility and then grouped various socioeconomic variables into three nonspatial factors: socioeconomic disadvantages, sociocultural barriers, and high healthcare needs. The authors proposed two kinds of shortage areas including areas of poor spatial access to primary care (with the combination of spatial access and high healthcare needs) and areas of disadvantaged population (with the combination of socioeconomic disadvantages and sociocultural barriers). This integration effectively delineates the areas short of primary care yet it does not consider the shortage areas of mammography screening services.

This research aims to develop an integrated approach to decide whether an area is short of mammography access. First, it uses the Gaussian 2SFCA to measure spatial accessibility between women (ages≥40) and mammography facilities in a Geographic Information Systems (GIS) environment. Second, it merges socioeconomic variables into three nonspatial factors to reflect the nonspatial barriers to access mammography facilities using factor analysis. Finally, it integrates spatial and nonspatial factors to identify the areas short of mammography access as well as their priorities. This approach may help the DHHS and the state health departments to designate shortage areas. Areas with higher priorities suggest more severe deprivation of mammography access. The approach can be easily adopted to identify factors that are responsible for poor access, which helps the health departments develop programs based on available resources.

STUDY AREA AND DATA

This report designates the mammography shortage areas in Michigan. Michigan is an appropriate study area because it includes both the densely populated metropolitan Detroit and sparsely populated rural regions. The selection of this area is also supported by previous studies. Dai (2010) reported that areas short of mammography facilities in metropolitan Detroit were associated with higher risks of late-stage diagnosis for breast cancer. Meliker et al. (2009) found urban areas had more significant clusters of early-stage breast cancer than rural regions in Michigan. Therefore, it is critical to identify the areas short of mammography access in Michigan in order to develop intervention and prevention accordingly.

Data pertaining to the addresses of 326 certified mammography facilities (locations in 2009) is compiled from the US Food and Drug Administration (USFDA, 2009). Each facility's coordinates (longitude and latitude) are collected from a private vendor named the ReferenceUSA. The vendor routinely updates its database and has been a reliable resource for research (e.g., Dai, 2010; Raja, Ma, & Yadav, 2008). Census 2000 Summary File 3 at census block group level and census tract level from the US Census Bureau are used to estimate the demographic and socioeconomic structures. It is admitted that the mammography facilities may change after the census was collected in 2000. Therefore, interpreting the results requires cautions and more recent census data sets are warranted once available to examine the change of the designated shortage areas.

SPATIAL ACCESS TO MAMMOGRAPHY FACILITIES IN MICHIGAN

The spatial accessibility measure relies on the Gaussian 2SFCA (Dai, 2010). Some studies used shortest travel time to the nearest mammography facility (e.g., McLafferty & Wang, 2009; Wang, McLafferty, Escamilla, & Luo, 2008) or average time to the five closest facilities (e.g., Tarlov, Zenk, Campbell, Warnecke, & Block, 2008). Such measures consider the availability of mammography screening resources but do not consider the interactions between supplies and demands—competition between facilities for a client and competition between clients for a facility (Luo & Wang, 2003; Wang & Luo, 2005). The previous research (Dai, 2010) has proven that the Gaussian 2SFCA performs better than the travel time to the closest facility in accounting for the spatial interactions. For each census tract, the Gaussian 2SFCA calculates a numerical value that represents the ratio of the local supplies of mammography facilities to the local demands (10,000 women with ages equal to or older than 40 years) for screening services. This research measures both supplies and demands in a search window within a fixed travel time (i.e., 30 minutes). A higher value using this measure represents a higher ratio of supplies to demands, and thus suggests a better access. For more details, see Dai (2010).

Population weighted centroids based on census block data are used to represent census tracts because they are more accurate than geographic centroids to reveal population unevenness (Dai, 2010; Luo & Wang, 2003). Travel time is estimated using the Network Analyst tool in ArcGIS 9.3 (Environmental Systems Research Institute, Inc., Redlands, CA). It simulates the shortest travel time through the road network using speed limits as the travel impedance. Although actual travel time may increase due to traffic congestion, taking public transits, or other factors, the estimated travel time along road network has been effectively used in research (e.g., Luo & Qi, 2009; McLafferty & Wang, 2009) to reflect the travel barrier.

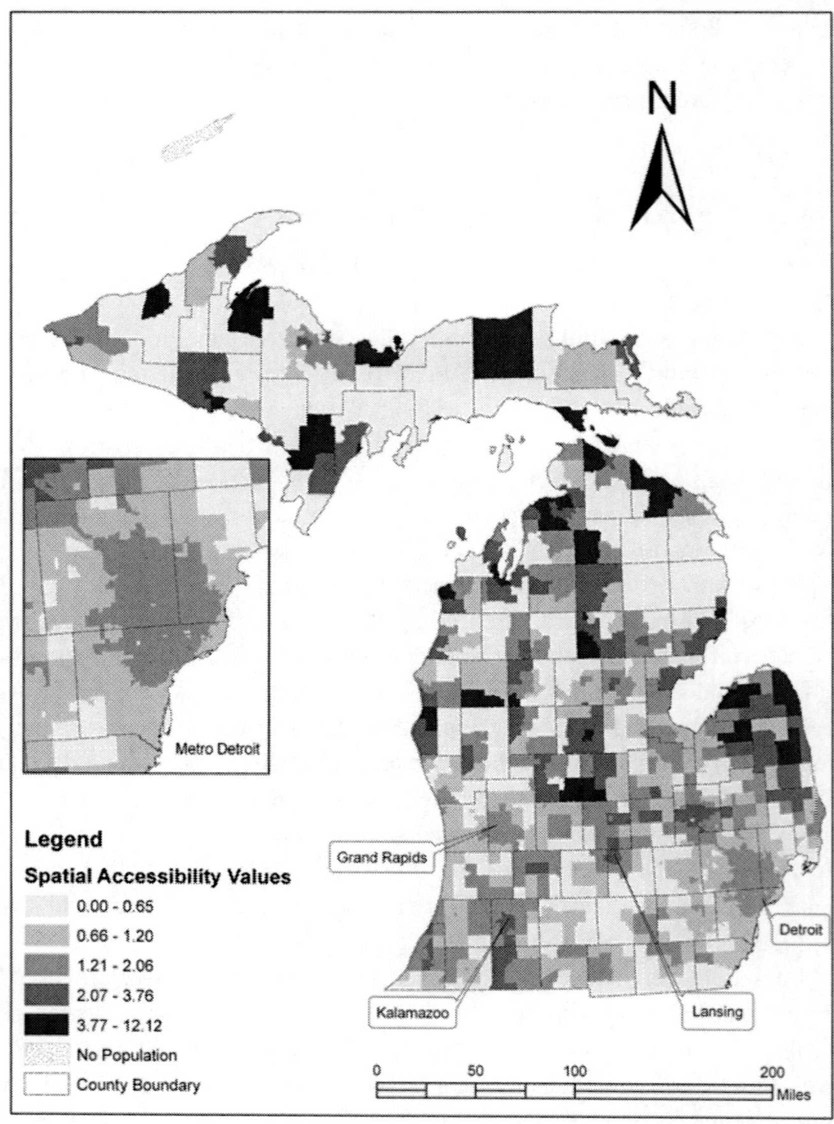

Figure 1. Spatial accessibility to mammography facilities (travel range is 30 min.).

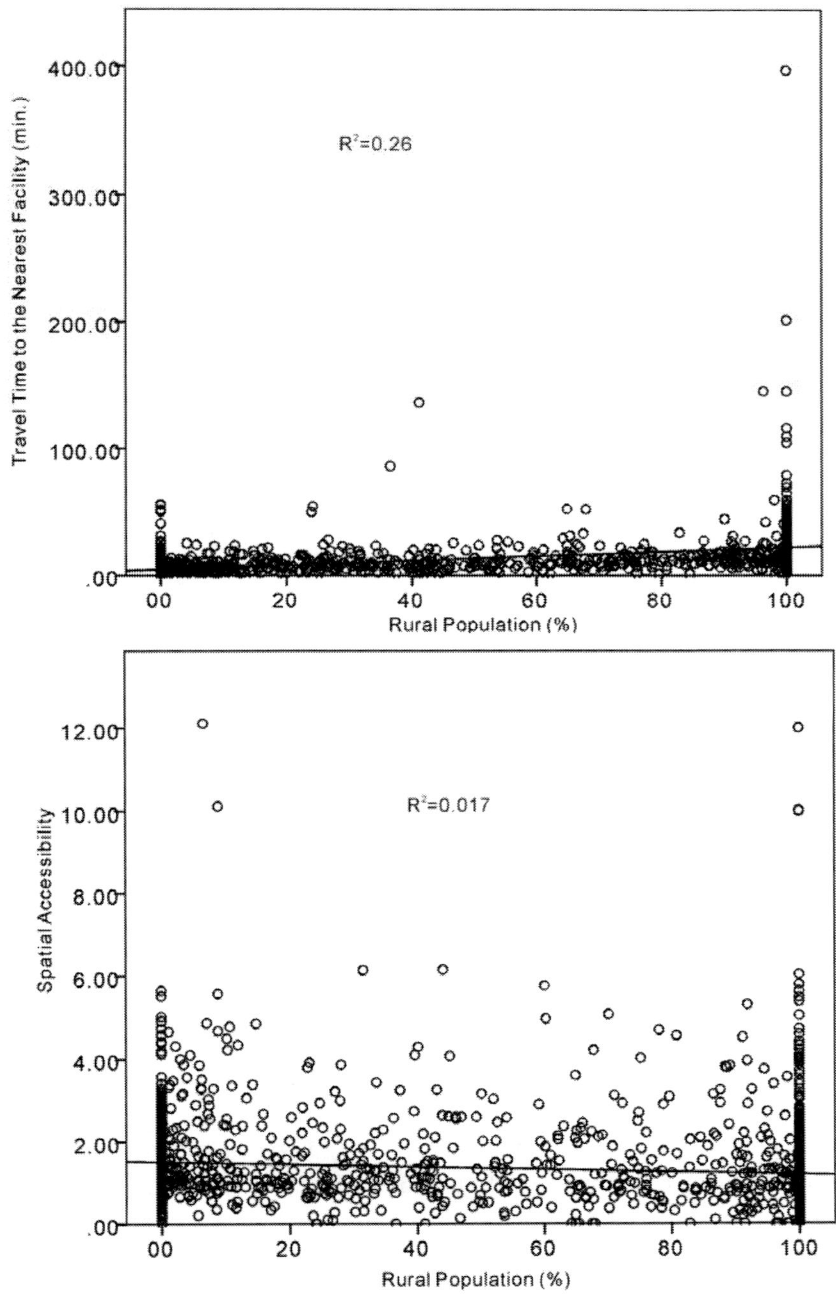

Figure 2. Rural-uran disparities in spaital accessbiltiy to mammography facilities.

Figure 1 shows an apparent geographic variation in mammography access in Michigan which favors urban and suburban residents. The accessibility values indicate the number of mammography facilities available to every 10,000 women (ages≥40 years) at each census tract. A previous research (Elkin et al., 2010) suggested that areas with a capacity of about 1.2 machines per 10,000 women (ages≥40) required to achieve a 70% screening rate, a goal proposed in Healthy People 2010 (2000). Based on this criterion, Upper Peninsula and northeast region of the Lower Peninsula are very deprived in accessing mammography facilities. Urban and suburban areas (e.g., Detroit and Grant Rapids) enjoy better access than most of the rural areas. This observation is consistent with the apparent urban-rural gradient (see Figure 2). In urban areas where their percentages of rural population are 0, the average travel time to the closest facility is 4.57 minutes and the average spatial accessibility score is 1.48. On the contrary, remote areas where their percentages of rural population are 100% have the average travel time of 24.32 minutes to the nearest facility and the average spatial accessibility score of 1.13.

NONSPATIAL ACCESS TO MAMMOGRAPHY FACILITIES

In addition to geographic barriers, access to screening mammography is highly related to nonspatial factors (age, income, ethnicity, and other the socioeconomic status of women. Previous studies (Field et al., 2005; Lian, Jeffe, & Schootman, 2008; MacKinnon et al., 2007) have shown that low-income women and racial and ethnic minorities may be disadvantaged in accessing mammography facilities. Therefore, it is critical to consider the nonspatial factors in evaluating mammography accessibility. In line with previous studies (Field, 2000; Goovaerts, 2005; Wang & Luo, 2005) as well as the guidelines from the DHHS for designating HPSAs, this research employed 15 variables based on the Census 2000 Summary File 3 at the census tract level. These variables include eligible women (40+), black population, rural population, linguistically isolated households, carless households, population without high-school diploma, population below poverty line, unemployed population, female headed households, professional and managerial jobs, home ownership, households with more than one occupant per room, median income, median housing value, and median gross rent. All variables are measured by percentage except the last three in US dollars. This study considers only African Americans because they predominate in Michigan

(14.21%) compared to other minorities (5.63%). The 15 variables provide a comprehensive description of the socioeconomic status in a census tract, yet the correlations between some variables make it difficult to interpret the deprivation of a neighborhood. For example, neighborhoods with lower education levels generally have lower proportions of professional and managerial jobs. To facilitate the interpretation of nonspatial barriers to access mammography, this research consolidates the 15 variables into three factors using factor analysis (Griffith & Amrhein, 1997; Wang, 2006).

Factor analysis is employed to remove the highly correlated variables and to replace them with a smaller number of uncorrelated variables. Factor analysis begins with principal component analysis (PCA). PCA finds a combination of variables (i.e., a factor) that accounts for as much as variation in the original variables as possible. It then finds another factor that is uncorrelated with the previous factor and accounts for as much of the remaining variation as possible. The process continues until it identifies as many factors as original variables. Each factor is associated with an eigenvalue explaining the variance it captures in the original data. Based on literature (Griffith & Amrhein, 1997), factor analysis then retains any factors with eigenvalues greater than one to represent the original variables. Consequently, factor analysis uses a few uncorrelated components to replace the original variables and accounts for the most of the variance of the original data. Compared to PCA preserving all information, factor analysis reduces the number of variables, thus making it easy to interpret the nonspatial barriers to access mammography facilities. Besides, it has been an effective tool in health studies (e.g., Goovaerts, 2005; Wang et al., 2008). Using factor analysis, this study retains three factors capturing 69.36% of the variation in the original variables (see Table 1), which are explained below.

Factor 1 represents socioeconomic disadvantages of a neighborhood. It captures seven variables (female headed households, carless households, black population, population below poverty line, unemployment population, housing ownership, and rural population), and is positively correlated with the first five variables. A higher factor 1 score reflects a more socioeconomically deprived neighborhood (e.g., a higher unemployment rate and a higher poverty rate). Figure 3 shows the spatial distribution of socioeconomic disadvantages in Michigan. It suggests that areas with high socioeconomic barriers (high scores or high socioeconomic disadvantages) are concentrated in urban centers. In contrast, areas with low socioeconomic barriers (low scores or low socioeconomic disadvantages) are located mostly in suburbs and rural communities.

Table 1. Rotated factor structure[a] of the socioeconomic variables

	Factor1	Factor2	Factor3
Female headed household (%)	*0.888*	-0.221	0.039
Carless household (%)	*0.832*	-0.285	0.121
Black population (%)	*0.816*	-0.186	-0.023
Population below poverty (%)	*0.727*	-0.416	0.323
Unemployment (%)	*0.664*	-0.461	0.067
Housing ownership (%)	*-0.712*	0.128	-0.354
Rural population (%)	*-0.605*	-0.450	-0.195
Professional and managerial job (%)	*-0.124*	*0.869*	-0.161
Median housing value	-0.279	*0.815*	-0.103
Median income	-0.431	*0.769*	-0.162
Median gross rent	-0.078	*0.666*	0.089
Population without high-school degree (%)	0.481	*-0.617*	0.313
Linguistic isolation (%)	0.084	0.118	*0.781*
Room with over one occupant (%)	0.427	-0.264	*0.657*
Female population (40+) (%)	-0.028	0.148	*-0.706*
% of variance explained	46.14	13.87	9.35

Note: [a]Rotation method is varimax with Kaiser Normalization in order to maximize the loading of the variables on one factor and minimize the loadings on the other two factors.

Values in italics suggest the major loading of a variable on a factor among the three factors.

Factor 2 reflects high social status of a neighborhood. It represents five variables (professional and managerial jobs, median housing value, median income, median gross rent, and population without high-school diploma), and is positively correlated with the first four variables. A higher factor 2 score represents a neighborhood with higher social status (e.g., a higher percentage of professional and managerial jobs and a higher income level). Figure 4 shows the spatial distribution of social status in Michigan. The figure shows that areas with high social status (high scores) are located mostly in the northwest suburbs of Detroit, as well as the suburbs in other cities (e.g., Lansing, Kalamazoo, and Grand Rapids). In addition, some areas near the Michigan Thumb region and the northwestern corner of the Lower Peninsula have high social status as well. On the contrary, areas with low social status (low scores) are present in the Upper Peninsula and the rural areas in the Lower Peninsula.

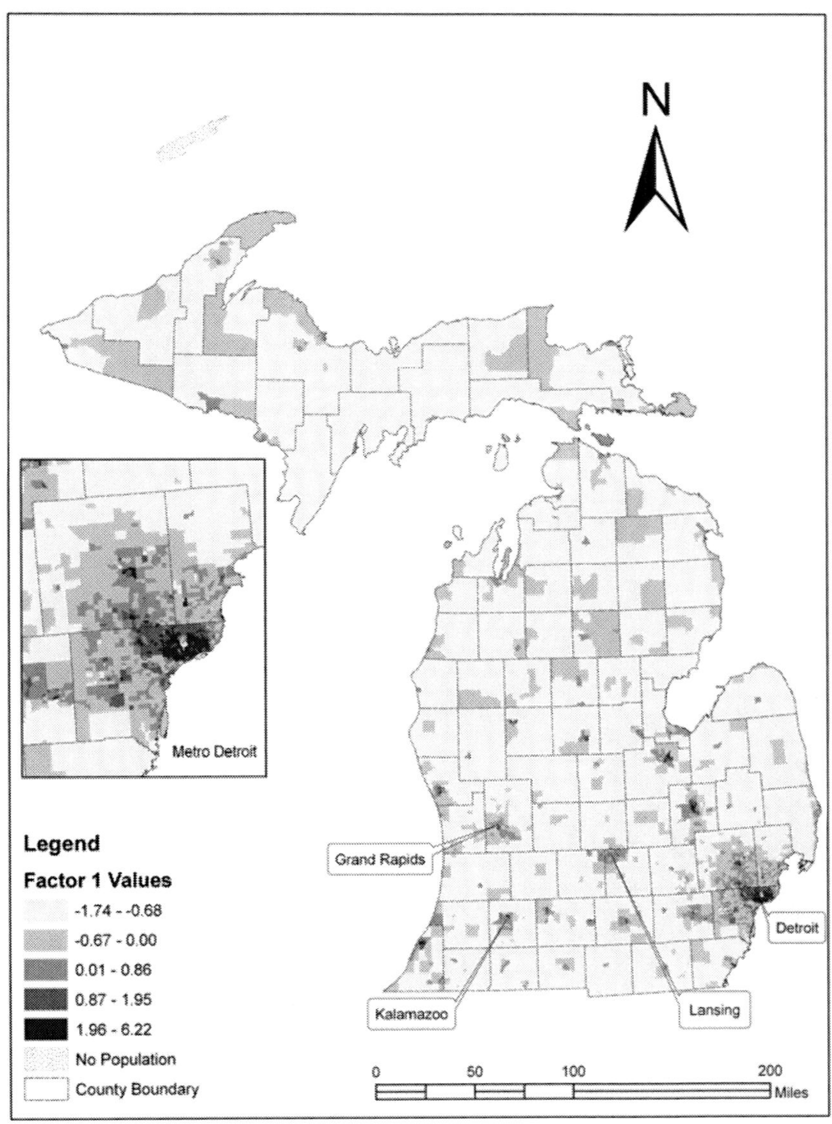

Figure 3. Socioeconomic disadvantages (Factor 1).

Factor 3 represents the high needs of mammography screening services. It reflects mainly three variables including linguistically isolated households, households with more than one person per room, and female population (ages≥40). Factor 3 is positively correlated with the first two and indicates two important populations. Neighborhoods with high factor 3 scores indicate strong linguistic isolation. Studies (Baron et al., 2008; Coronado, Thompson, & Chen, 2009) suggested that women with linguistic barriers were less likely to have routine access to mammography screening.

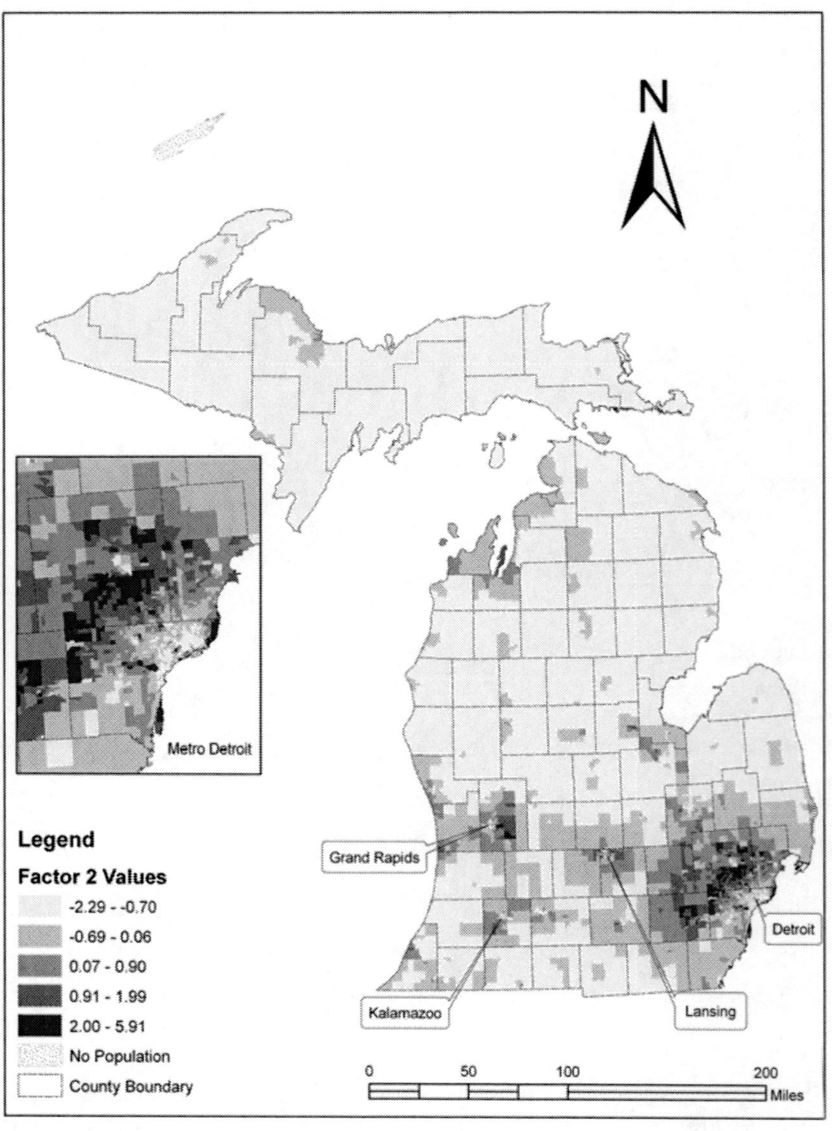

Figure 4. High social status (Factor 2).

These areas therefore reflect high linguistic needs to access screening services. On the contrary, neighborhoods with lower factor 3 scores suggest higher percentages of female population (ages≥40) despite low linguistic barriers. These areas reflect high age needs for screening services given the large percentages of the residing eligible female population (ages≥40). Therefore, areas with either high or low factor 3 scores reflect the high screening needs. Figure 5 suggests that areas with high linguistic needs of screening services (very high scores) are located in urban centers (e.g., Detroit or Grand Rapids). Areas with high age needs are mainly in the Upper Peninsula and the northern regions of the Lower Peninsula.

Integrating Spatial and Nonspatial Factors to Evaluate Mammography Access in Michigan

To identify the areas short of mammography access, this research integrates the spatial accessibility measure and the three nonspatial factors because all of them are important to mammography access. Spatial accessibility measure serves as the primary factor as long travel time makes it difficult to receive routine screening services. Using 1.2 as the threshold as recommended in a research (Elkin et al., 2010), this study classifies the census tracts into three categories: absolute shortage (spatial accessibility is 0), moderate shortage (spatial accessibility between 0 and 1.2), and no shortage (spatial accessibility is greater than or equal to 1.2). For nonspatial factors, very poor access is associated with a very high factor 1 score (high socioeconomic disadvantages), a very low factor 2 score (low social status), and a very low (high age needs) or very high (high linguistic needs) factor 3 score. Therefore, the shortage areas are defined as follows with decreasing priorities for intervention:

Area 1 (top priority): census tracts with the spatial accessibility scores equal to zero regardless of the nonspatial factors.

Area 2 (high priority): census tracts with the spatial accessibility scores greater than zero but less than 1.2, if at least one of the three nonspatial factors is disadvantaged. Wang and Luo (2005) defined a score higher than one standard deviation above its mean value as a shortage area. Following this rule and the characteristics of the three factors in this study, factor 1 would be disadvantaged if it scores one standard deviation above its mean. Similarly, factor 2 would be disadvantaged if it scores one standard deviation below its mean, and factor 3 would be disadvantaged if it scores one standard deviation either above or below its mean value.

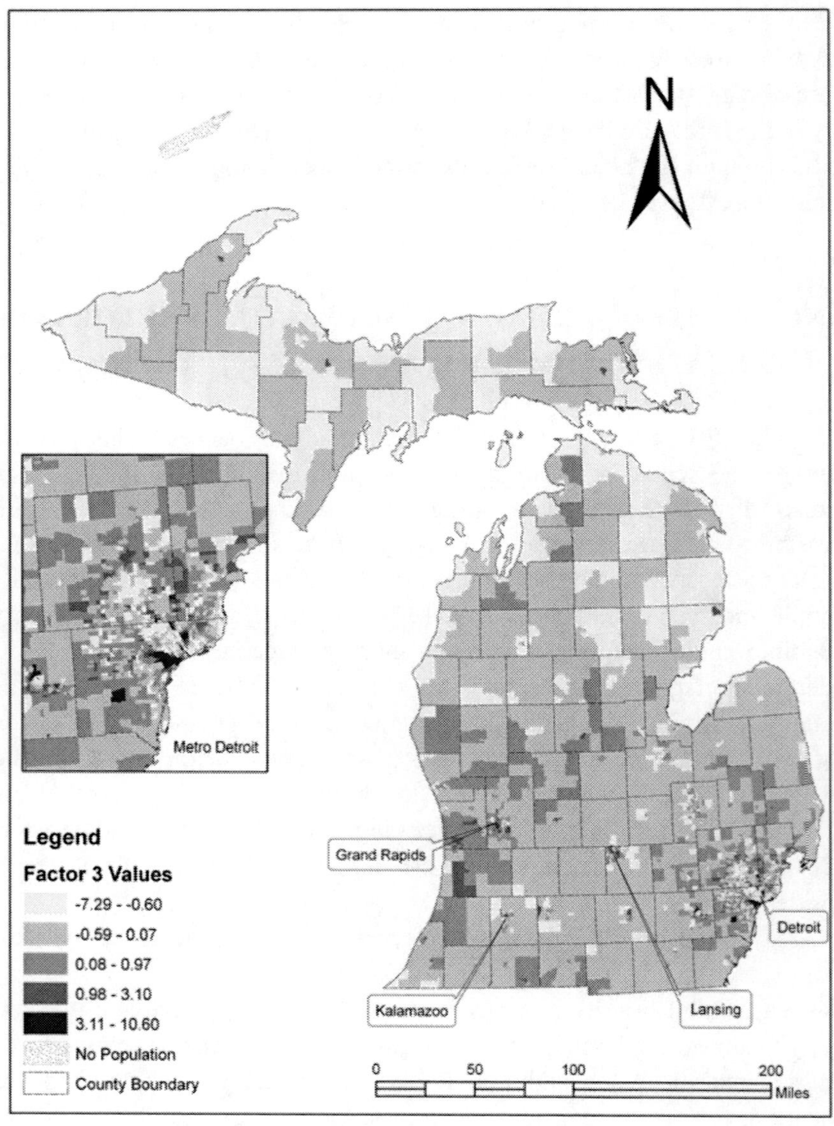

Figure 5. High screening needs (Factor 3).

Area 3 (medium priority): census tracts with the spatial accessibility scores greater than zero but less than 1.2, if none of the three nonspatial factors is disadvantaged.

Area 4 (low priority): census tracts with the spatial accessibility scores greater than or equal to 1.2, if at least one of the three nonspatial factors is disadvantaged.

Area 5 (lowest priority): census tracts with the spatial accessibility scores greater than or equal to 1.2, if none of the three nonspatial factors is disadvantaged.

Figure 6 presents the mammography shortage areas using this integrated approach. Area 1 exhibits the most deprived areas short of mammography facilities. These areas have no mammography facilities within a driving range of 30 minutes and shall receive the highest priority for improving mammography accessibility. Area 2 suggests that a census tract has poor spatial access and also has at least one disadvantaged nonspatial factor. As can be seen, these tracts are located mostly in the Upper Peninsula, as well as central and southern Michigan in the Lower Peninsula. In metropolitan Detroit, such tracts are mostly located in the southwest and northeast suburbs. Area 3 indicates that a census tract has poor spatial access without disadvantaged nonspatial factors. These areas are mostly in close proximity to large cities in the Lower Peninsula. Areas 4 and 5 suggest that tracts have high spatial access to mammography facilities. Area 4 is deprived because of one or more disadvantaged nonspatial factors, which can be seen mostly in urban centers.

To evaluate the sensitivity of this classification, this research explores two additional scenarios. In scenario 2, the criterion for nonspatial factors is that at least two factors are disadvantaged in order to change a tract's priority. For instance, area 2 suggests that tracts have poor spatial access and have two or three disadvantaged nonspatial factors. Figure 7 shows the mammography shortage areas in scenario 2. Tracts in areas 2 and 4 apparently decrease compared to the first scenario (see Figure 5). In scenario 3, the criterion is that all three nonspatial factors must be disadvantaged in order to change a tract's priority. As mapped in Figure 8, tracts in areas 2 and 4 significantly decrease compared to scenarios 1 and 2. Only three census tracts are in area 2: one large tract is in the southwest Detroit, and the other two are located in the central city of Detroit. Area 4 is mainly in Detroit as well where residents have poor nonspatial access to mammography facilities despite their rich spatial access. Table 2 summarizes the population living in the designated shortage areas. In general, more than 40% of women (ages$\geq$40) in Michigan live in areas short of spatial access to mammography facilities. Approximate 69,551 eligible women cannot reach any mammography services within a driving range of 30 minutes.

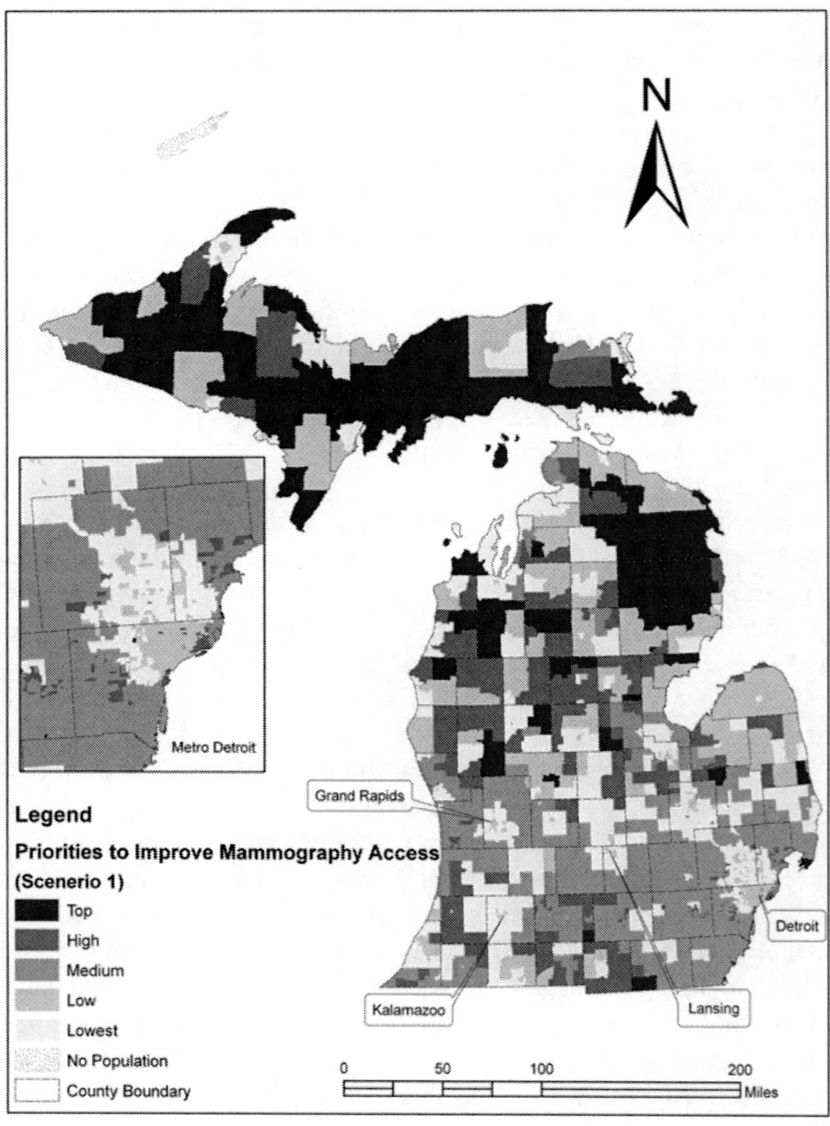

Figure 6. Designated mammography shortage areas in Michigan in the first scenario.

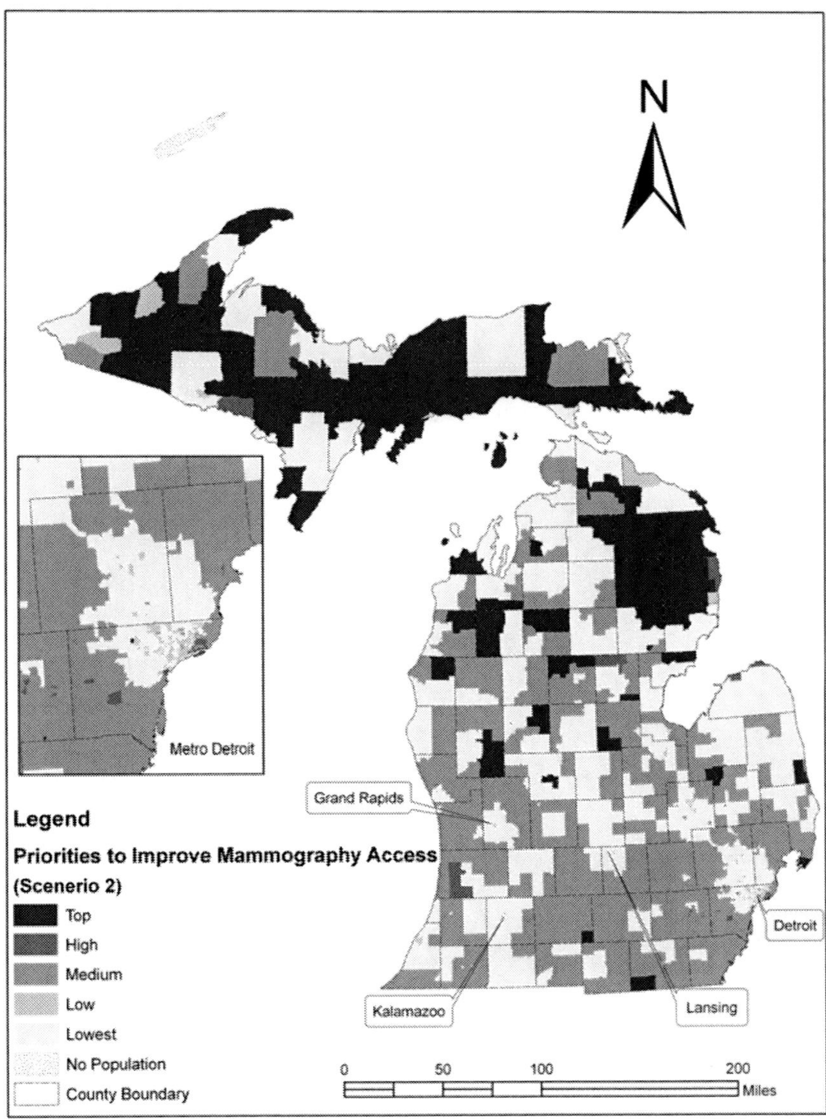

Figure 7. Designated mammography shortage areas in Michigan in the second scenario.

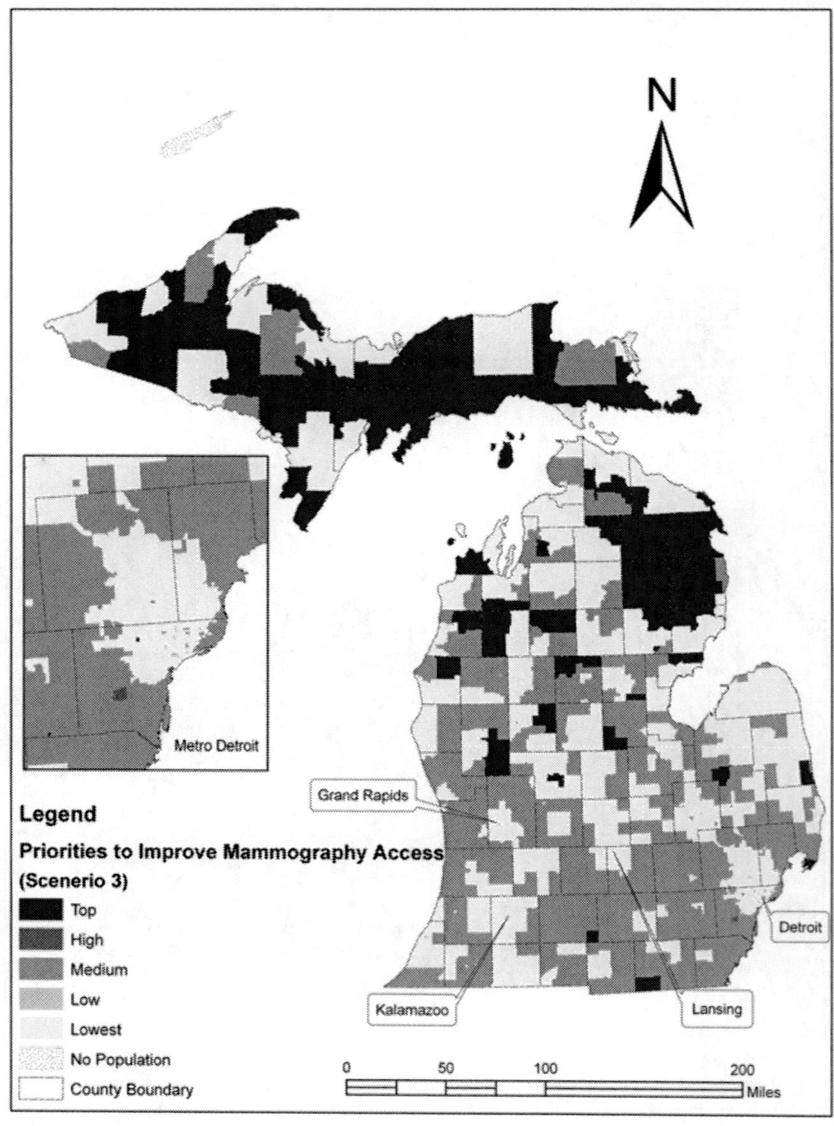

Figure 8. Designated mammography shortage areas in Michigan in the third scenario.

Table 2. Summary of the population living in the designated shortage areas

Scenerio	Rank	Spatial Access	Disadvantaged nonspatial factors (#)	Tract (#)	Tract (%)	Area (km²)	Area (%)	Women (#)	Women (%)
	1	0		95	3.50	39,978.16	26.67	69,551	3.07
	2	(0, 1.2)	At least one factor	242	8.93	25,051.95	16.71	168,199	7.43
1	3	(0, 1.2)	Others	754	27.81	27,952.06	18.64	679,731	30.01
	4	[1.2, 12.12]	At least one factor	623	22.98	29,632.67	19.77	429,967	18.98
	5	[1.2, 12.12]	Others	997	36.78	27,308.15	18.21	917,428	40.51
	1	0		95	3.50	39,978.16	26.67	69,551	3.07
	2	(0, 1.2)	At least two factors	39	1.44	1,436.93	0.96	19,671	0.87
2	3	(0, 1.2)	Others	957	35.30	51,567.08	34.40	828,259	36.57
	4	[1.2, 12.12]	At least two factors	156	5.75	1,632.25	1.09	79,911	3.53
	5	[1.2, 12.12]	Others	1,464	54.00	55,308.57	36.89	1,267,484	55.96
	1	0		95	3.50	39,978.16	26.67	69,551	3.07
	2	(0, 1.2)	All three factors	3	0.11	25.57	0.02	1,361	0.06
3	3	(0, 1.2)	Others	993	36.63	52,978.45	35.34	846,569	37.38
	4	[1.2, 12.12]	All three factors	13	0.48	17.29	0.01	4,979	0.22
	5	[1.2, 12.12]	Others	1,607	59.28	56,923.53	37.97	1,342,416	59.27
	Total			2,711	100%	149,923.00	100%	2,264,876	100%

Note: the maximum spatial accessiblity score is 12.12.

This integrated approach has a number of advantages. First, it provides a systematic depiction of mammography shortage areas by considering both spatial and nonspatial factors. As discussed in the introduction, mammography access is influenced by both spatial and nonspatial barriers. Long-distance traveling discourages women to seek mammography screening in time (Dinkelspiel, Chu, & Smith-Bindman, 2008; Tarlov et al., 2008; Zenk, Tarlov, & Sun, 2006). Women from low-income families or with linguistic barriers may hesitate to have screening services because of economic or cultural reasons even if they are close to screening facilities (Field et al., 2005; Lian et al., 2008; MacKinnon et al., 2007). This current approach uncovers the true disadvantages of each census tract from both spatial and nonspatial aspects. Second, this method assigns priorities to the census tracts. Once the true disadvantages of the census tracts are identified, they can be addressed accordingly. Areas with higher priorities suggest more severe deprivation of mammography access and shall receive more attention than other areas. Finally, this approach is flexible because it provides multiple scenarios to address mammography shortage. For example, if resources for intervention are limited, a tightened designation scheme may be used (e.g., scenario 3). The multiple scenarios give local health department personnel flexibility to develop programs based on available resources.

CONCLUSION

This research evaluates areas short of mammography access by consolidating spatial and nonspatial factors. First, it uses a Gaussian-based two step floating catchment area method to quantify spatial accessibility in a GIS environment. Second, it generates three socioeconomic factors affecting the nonspatial access to mammography screening using factor analysis. Finally, it integrates the spatial and nonspatial factors into one evaluation scheme and prioritizes the shortage areas. Such integration can help health professionals assess the needs (e.g., spatial needs, linguistic needs, or educational needs) in areas short of screening services, and deliver resources to the shortage areas according to their actual needs and their priorities.

In conclusion, identifying areas short of mammography screening services is an important step to understand the persistent disparities in breast cancer mobility and mortality. The current study proposes a systematic approach to evaluate the shortage areas as well as the corresponding needs. In light of the shortage of mammography access in Michigan, this research shows that the rural areas are likely to have poor spatial access to mammography services, calling for the increase of mammography availability in these remote regions. On the contrary, the concentration of nonspatial barriers in urbanized neighborhoods emphasizes the need for extensive education and screening programs specifically targeting the vulnerable urban residents in these places. The approach illustrated here can be easily adopted to help identify and communicate about factors that are responsible for poor mammography access, as well as understand their implications to breast cancer prevention and control.

REFERENCES

American Cancer Society. (2009). *Breast Cancer Facts and Figures 2009-2010*. Atlanta, GA: American Cancer Society, Inc.

Baron, R. C., Rimer, B. K., Coates, R. J., Kerner, J., Kalra, G. P., Melillo, S., et al. (2008). Client-directed interventions to increase community access to breast, cervical, and colorectal cancer screening: a systematic review. *American Journal of Preventive Medicine, 35*(1S), S56-S66.

Barton, M. B. (2001). Screening mammography for women aged 40-49: Are we off the fence yet? *CMAJ, 164*(4), 498-499.

Breen, N., Cronin, K. A., Meissner, H. I., Taplin, S. H., Tangka, F. K., Tiro, J. A., et al. (2007). Reported drop in mammography: Is this cause for concern? *Cancer, 109*(12), 2405-2409.

Cervigni, F., Suzuki, Y., Ishii, T., & Hata, A. (2008). Spatial accessibility to pediatric services. *Journal of Community Health, 33*, 444-448.

Coronado, G. D., Thompson, B., & Chen, L. (2009). Sociodemographic correlates of cancer screening services among hispanics and non-hispanic whites in a rural setting. *American Journal of Health Behavior, 33*(2), 181-191.

Cronan, T. A., Villalta, I., Gottfried, E., Vaden, Y., Ribas, M., & Conway, T. L. (2008). Predictors of mammography screening among ethnically diverse low-income women. *Journal of Women's Health, 17*(4), 527-537.

Dai, D. (2010). Black residental segregation, disparities in spatial access to health care facilities, and late-stage breast cancer diagnosis in metropolitan Detroit. *Health and Place, 16*, 1038-1052.

Dinkelspiel, E., Chu, P., & Smith-Bindman, R. (2008). Access to diagnostic mammography in the San Francisco Bay area. *Journal of Women's Health, 17*(5), 893-899.

Elkin, E. B., Ishill, N. M., Snow, J. G., Panageas, K. S., Bach, P. B., Liberman, L., et al. (2010). Geographic access and the use of screening mammography. *Medical Care, 48*(4), 349-356.

Field, K. (2000). Measuring the need for primary health care: an index of relative disadvantage. *Applied Geography, 20*, 305-332.

Field, T. S., Buist, D. S., Doubeni, C., Enger, S., Fouayzi, H., Hart, G., et al. (2005). Disparities and survival among breast cancer patients. *Journal of National Cancer Institute Monographs, 35*, 88-95.

Goovaerts, P. (2005). *Analysis and detection of health disparities using geostatistics and a space-time information system: the case of prostate cancer mortality in the United States, 1970 - 1994.* Paper presented at the GIS Planet 2005, Estorial, Portugal.

Griffith, D. A., & Amrhein, C. G. (1997). *Multivariate Statistical Analysis for Geographers*. Upper Saddle River, New Jersey: Prentice Hall.

Guagliardo, M. F. (2004). Spatial accessibility of primary care: concepts, methods and challenges. *International Journal of Health Geographics, 3*(3).

Institute of Medicine. (2003) *Fulfilling the potential of cancer prevention and early detection.* Washington DC: National Cancer Policy Board, Institute of Medicine of the National Academies.

Jackson, M. C., Davis, W. W., Waldron, W., McNeel, T. S., Pfeiffer, R., & Breen, N. (2009). Impact of geography on mammography use in California. *Cancer Causes & Control, 20*(8), 1339-1353.

Langford, M., & Higgs, G. (2006). Measuring potential access to primary healthcare services: the influence of alternative spatial representations of population. *The Professional Geographer, 58*(3), 294-306.

Lian, M., Jeffe, D. B., & Schootman, M. (2008). Racial and geographic differences in mammography screening in St. Louis City: A multilevel study. *Journal of Urban Health, 85*(5), 667-692.

Luo, W., & Qi, Y. (2009). An enhanced two-step floating catchment area (E2SFCA) method for measuring spatial accessibility to primary care physicians. *Health and Place, 15*(4), 1100-1107.

Luo, W., & Wang, F. (2003). Measures of spatial accessibility to health care in a GIS environment: synthesis and a case study in the Chicago region. *Environmental and Planning B: Planning and Design, 30*, 865-884.

MacKinnon, J. A., Duncan, R. C., Huang, Y., Lee, D. J., Fleming, L. E., Voti, L., et al. (2007). Detecting an association between socioeconomic status and late stage breast cancer using spatial analysis and area-based measures. *Cancer Epidemiology, Biomarkers and Prevention, 16*(4), 756-762.

McLafferty, S., & Wang, F. (2009). Rural reversal? Rural-urban disparities in late-stage cancer risk in Illinois. *Cancer, 115*, 2755-2764.

Meliker, J. R., Jacquez, G. M., Goovaerts, P., Copeland, G., & Yassine, M. (2009). Spatial cluster analysis of early stage breast cancer: a method for public health practice using cancer registry data. *Cancer Causes and Control.*

Raja, S., Ma, C., & Yadav, P. (2008). Beyond food deserts: Measuring and mapping racial disparities in neighborhood food environment. *Journal of Planning Education and Research, 27*, 469-482.

Tarlov, E., Zenk, S. N., Campbell, R. T., Warnecke, R. B., & Block, R. (2008). Characteristics of mammography facility locations and stage of breast cancer at diagnosis in Chicago. *Journal of Urban Health, 86*(2), 196-213.

US Department of Health and Human Services. (2000). *Healthy People 2010: Understanding and Improving Health.* Washington, DC. Available at http://www.healthpeople.gov/publications/. Last access on 8 October 2010.

US Food and Drug Administration. (2009). *Mammography Facilities.* Available at http://www.accessdata.fda.gov/scripts. Last access on 20 September 2009.

Wang, F. (2006). *Quantitative Methods and Applications in GIS.* Boca Raton, Florida: CRC Press.

Wang, F., & Luo, W. (2005). Assessing spatial and nonspatial factors for healthcare access: towards an integrated approach to defining health professional shortage areas. *Health and Place, 11*, 131-146.

Wang, F., McLafferty, S., Escamilla, V., & Luo, L. (2008). Late-stage breast cancer diagnosis and health care access in Illinois. *The Professional Geographer, 60*(1), 54-69.

Wells, K. J., & Roetzheim, R. G. (2007). Health disparities in receipt of screening mammography in Latinas: A critical review of recent literature. *Cancer Control, 14*(4), 369-379.

Zenk, S. N., Tarlov, E., & Sun, J. (2006). Spatial equity in facilities providing low- or no-fee screening mammography in Chicago neighborhoods. *Journal of Urban Health, 83*(2), 195-210.

In: Mammography:
Editors: A. Palmetti, R. Roux
ISBN 978-1-61470-589-5

Chapter 7

ACCESS TO MAMMOGRAPHY FACILITIES AND DETECTION OF BREAST CANCER BY SCREENING MAMMOGRAPHY: A GIS APPROACH

Selina Rahman[1,2*], James H. Price[2], Mark Dignan[4], Saleh Rahman[5], Peter S. Lindquist[3] and Timothy R. Jordan[2]

[1] Environmental Sciences Institute, Florida A and M University, Tallahassee, Florida

[2] Department of Health and Human Services, University of Toledo, OH, U. S.

[3] Department of Geography and Planning, University of Toledo, OH, U. S.

[4] Prevention Research Center, University of Kentucky, Lexington, Kentucky, U. S.

[5] Institute of Public Health, Florida A and M University, Tallahassee, Florida

[*] Email address: Selina.rahman@famu.edu

ABSTRACT

Objectives: The objective of the study was to examine the association between access to mammography facilities and utilization of screening mammography in an urban population.

Methods: Data on female breast cancer cases were obtained from an extensive mammography surveillance project. Distance to mammography facilities was measured by using GIS, which was followed by measuring geographical access to mammography facilities using Floating Catchment Area (FCA) Method (considering all available facilities within an arbitrary radius from the woman's residence by using Arc GIS 9.0 software).

Results: Of 2,024 women, 91.4% were Caucasian; age ranged from 25 to 98 years; most (95%) were non-Hispanic in origin. Logistic regression found age, family history, hormone replacement therapy, physician recommendation, and breast cancer stage at diagnosis to be significant predictors of having had a previous mammogram. Women having higher access to mammography facilities were less likely to have had a previous mammogram compared to women who had low access, considering all the facilities within 10 miles (OR=0.41, CI=0.22-0.76), 30 miles (OR=0.52, CI=0.29-0.91) and 40 miles (OR=0.51, CI=0.28-0.92) radiuses. *Conclusions:* Physical distance to mammography facilities does not necessarily predict utilization of mammogram and greater access does not assure greater utilizations, due to constraints imposed by socio economic and cultural barriers. Future studies should focus on measuring access to mammography facilities capturing a broader dimension of access considering qualitative aspect of facilities, as well as other travel impedances.

Keywords: Mammography, GIS, access, distance, breast cancer.

INTRODUCTION

Breast cancer is one of the leading causes of death among women in the United States. The American Cancer Society estimated that 178,480 new cases and 40,460 deaths from breast cancer occurred among women in the United States in 2007 (American Cancer Society [ACS], 2007). Due to a lack of primary prevention of breast cancer, breast cancer mortality and morbidity reduction depends on secondary prevention, chiefly through screening mammography. Several randomized trials as well as population-based screening evaluations have indicated that early detection of breast cancer through screening mammography improves treatment options, the likelihood of successful treatment, and improved survival (William, Holladay, and Sheikh 2003; Taber et al., 2003; Humphrey, Helfand, Chan, and Woolf, 2002; Duffy, Tabar, and Chen, 2002). A rise in mammography utilization is suggested by the observed trends (1987-1999) of an increase in breast cancer incidence confined to early stage breast cancer (Howe, et al., 2001; Edwards, et al., 2002; Blanchard, et al. 2004). A significant and substantial reduction in female breast cancer mortality has been observed in recent years because of screening mammography (Smith, et al., 2003; Duffy et al., 2006). However, the mortality rate from breast cancer is still too high, even though screening rates have increased and mortality decreased somewhat. The Healthy People 2010 target is 22.3 deaths per 100,000 women, but according to the American Cancer Society data the death rate is 26 per 100,000 women in 2007 (ACS, 2007).

Several researchers have explored barriers to obtaining mammograms, including the physical distance to mammography facilities and other barriers (Ann, Ronald, Raymond, and Gilligan, 2001; Jilda, Hyndman, and Holman, 2000a; Jilda, Hyndman, and Holman, 2000b). Understanding the geographical and social connections between the utilization of mammography and the locations of mammography facilities is critically important for developing effective programs to reduce breast cancer mortality. Health Education Promotion programs designed to increase mammography screening and produce subsequent reduction in breast cancer mortality may have opportunities to improve their effectiveness if they are able take barriers such as geographic distance to screening services into consideration. Health care decisions are strongly influenced by the type and quality of services available in the local area and the distance, time, cost, and ease of traveling to reach those services (Goodman, Fisher, Stukel, and Chang, 1997; Haynes, Bentham, Lovett, and Gale, 1999; Joseph and Phillips, 1984; Croner, Sperling, and Broome, 1996; Fortney, Rost, and Warren, 2003). The term 'spatial accessibility' is gaining more and more attention in the health care geography literature (Khan and Bhardwaj, 1994; Luo, 2004; Luo and Wang, 2003), which is a combination of dimensions of accessibility (travel impedance between patients and service points, that is measured in units of distance or travel time), and availability (refers to the number of local service locations from which a patient can choose). In this study, we focused on measuring access to mammogram facility by using GIS, considering both accessibility and availability dimensions. We also examined whether access to mammography facilities and other demographic variables influence utilization of mammography.

Methods

Data Collection

The data for this study were obtained from the Colorado Mammography Project (CMAP). CMAP was a National Cancer Institute funded project that was in operation from 1994-2004. CMAP was one member of a seven-site consortium, and obtained data on mammograms from approximately half of all mammography facilities in the six-county Denver metropolitan area of Colorado. For this study, information on mammograms for women from 1999-2001 was analyzed. The CMAP database included demographic data (age, race/ethnicity, education, and insurance status), data on mammogram results, previous mammogram history, family history, use of hormone replacement therapy, physician recommendation, and the zip codes of women's residences. Addresses of mammography facilities participating in CMAP were obtained for this study from the Colorado Department of Public Health and Environment. There were 46 facilities on the list that were operating during the time period (1999-2001) and were considered as the possible facilities that women might use to obtain a mammogram.

Calculation of Access to Mammography Facility

We used the "Floating catchment area" (FCA) method by Luo and Wang (2004) to calculate access, that considered all available facilities within an arbitrary radius around a woman's address. Forty-six mammography facilities were geocoded using the ArcGIS System and placed in a separate file. Zip code centroids were obtained from a Zip code polygon file and compared to the database of patients. All Zip code centroids that had no patients from the sample were discarded, and then the numbers of patients were summed for each Zip code centroid and placed in a separate file. Mammography facility points and Zip code centroid points were connected to the regional street and highway network. Point-to-Point mileages were computed in a separate shortest path utility embedded within the GIS. The mileages were outputted in the form of a distance matrix. The distance matrix between Zip code centroids and mammography facilities was then imported into an Excel spreadsheet.

Minimum distance that a woman would be willing to travel to get to a mammogram was considered 10, 20, 30, 40, or, 50 miles and following operations were performed for each of these arbitrary radius. For each specified radius, the number of women among all Zip codes within the specified radius was summed for each of the 46 mammography facilities identified within the study area. Then the inverse of these sums were computed to calculate the availability of that facility. Now, for each woman's Zip code within a specified radius, the availability for all facilities was summed to obtain the FCA index, representing her access to mammogram facility. Finally, indices for five different arbitrary radii 10, 20, 30, 40, and 50 miles were computed to calculate access to mammography facility.

Statistical Analysis to Examine Relationship between the Variables

To further explore the association between the variables, logistic regressionwas performed. The dependent variable entered into the logistic model was whether the woman has had a previous mammogram or not (coded as yes=1 and No=0). Women who had a previous record of mammogram in the CMAP database or answered, "yes" on their patient information form when asked about their previous mammogram history at their index examination were considered as having had a previous mammogram (Figure 1 displays the distribution of the study population that did not have a previous mammogram in the six county areas).

A series of categorical variables were created and entered into the logistic model such as, age, race/ethnicity, education, insurance status, family history, hormone replacement therapy, physician recommendation, and breast cancer stage at diagnosis along with access to mammography facilities. Among the independent variables, the 'physician recommendation' variable was divided into two broad categories: 'diagnostic' that included all the diagnostic procedures (such as, biopsy, needle localization, and ultrasound) and 'evaluative' that included the rest of the categories, such as, follow up, physical examination, surgical consultation etc. Breast cancer stage at diagnosis was also condensed into two categories: non-advanced breast cancer stage at diagnosis included carcinoma *in situ*, and localized tumors, which are malignant and invasive but confined to the organ of origin; and advanced stage of breast cancer at diagnosis included regional neoplasm that have extended beyond the organ of origin into surrounding tissues, involving regional lymph nodes, or both, and distant tumors that have spread to remote parts of the body from the primary site.

With the access ratio for five different radii (such as, 10 miles, 20 miles, 30 miles, 40 miles, and 50 miles) five different logistic regression models were developed. Both univariate and multivariate analyses were conducted and on the basis of analysis of maximum likelihood estimates, significant interaction terms were identified and there was no significant interaction between the variables.

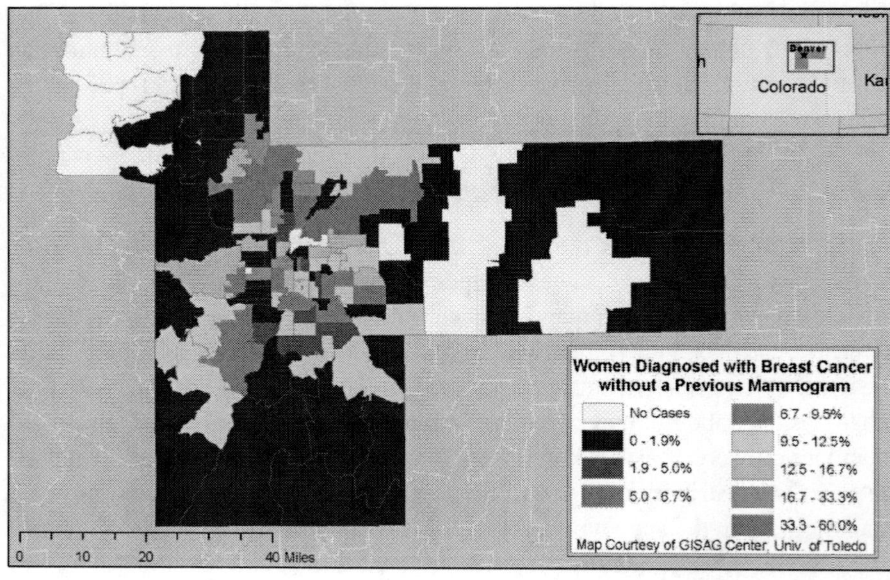

Figure 1. Distribution of Population Who did not have had a Previous Mammogram (by Zip Code).

Results

Demographic Characteristics

The data from the Colorado Cancer Registry included 2042 individuals diagnosed with breast cancer during the period of 1999 to 2001. Descriptive statistics for the study population are summarized in Table 1.

The breast cancer cases ranged in age from 25 to 98 years with 30% being 50-59 years of age and nearly all were Caucasian (91%). Twenty one percent reported having Medicaid and/or Medicare and 78% also had private insurance.

Among those with data on family history, 17% had a positive family history of breast cancer. Among those with data on hormone replacement therapy, 42% were on hormone replacement therapy at the time of the initial mammogram. Nearly all (91%) of the women in the database had a previous mammogram.

Table 1. Characteristics of the Study Population

Factors	Number (N=2042)	Percentage (%)
Age		
Below 40 years	121	6
40-49	503	24
50-59	609	30
60-69	364	18
70 years and above	445	22
Race/Ethnicity		
White	1811	91
Black	45	2
Asian	17	<1
American Indians and others	5	<1
Hispanic	104	5
Ethnicity		
Hispanic	104	5
Non Hispanic	1898	95
Education		
Less than High School Graduate	46	6
High School Graduate	198	26
Some College	251	32
College, or Post Graduate	280	36
Insurance Status		
Medicaid and/or Medicare	392	21
No Insurance	15	<1
Other (Private insurance, managed care and others)	1417	78
Stage of Breast Cancer		
In situ	320	16
Localized	1080	56
Regional	498	26
Direct	32	2
Previous mammogram		
Yes	1560	91

Table 1. Continued

Factors	Number (N=2042)	Percentage (%)
No	155	9
Family History		
Yes	190	17
No	953	83
Hormone replacement therapy		
Yes	440	42
No	608	58
Physician Recommendation		
Diagnostic	497	46
Evaluative	585	54

Note. Totals do not add to 2042 because of missing values.
Percentage calculated based on the non-missing values.

Table 2 presents the odds ratios for the factors influencing having had a previous mammogram. Access to mammography facilities was negatively associated with having had a previous mammogram in the adjusted model developed for 10 miles, 30 miles, and 40 miles radius. Women who had greater access to mammography facilities were 59% less likely and women who had medium access to such facilities were 58% less likely respectively of having had a previous mammogram, compared to women who had low access to mammography facilities; and these findings were significant in both the crude and adjusted models for the 10 miles radius measure.

Table 2. OR for Factors Predicting Women who had a Previous Mammogram

Factors	Crude OR	95% CI	Adjusted OR	95% CI
Age Group				
Below 40 years	0.13	0.07-0.22*	0.11	0.06-0.22*
40-49	*1.00*		1.00	
50-59	3.24	1.81-5.80*	1.63	0.80-3.32
60-69	2.79	1.44-5.40*	1.72	0.77-3.90
70 years and above	0.73	0.47-1.14	1.02	0.50-2.09
Race/Ethnicity				
White	*1.00*		*1.00*	
Black	0.45	0.18-1.10	0.68	0.20-2.19
Asian	1.57	0.21-11.89	2.75	0.21-35.65
Factors	Crude OR	95% CI	Adjusted OR	95% CI

Hispanic		0.37	0.21-0.66*	0.51	0.06-4.69
Ethnicity					
Hispanic		*1.00*		*1.00*	
Non Hispanic		2.03	1.17-3.52*	1.55	0.19-12.82
Education					
Less than High School Graduate		*1.00*		*1.00*	
High School Graduate		0.33	0.20-0.54*	0.66	0.34-1.26
Some College		0.32	0.21-0.51*	0.65	0.36-1.19
College, or Post Graduate		0.38	0.24-0.60*	0.82	0.44-1.51
Insurance Status					
Medicaid and/or Medicare		0.38	0.19-0.75*	0.48	0.20-1.17
No insurance		*1.00*		*1.00*	
Other (Private insurance, managed care and others)		0.64	0.34-1.22	0.95	0.43-2.13
Family History					
Yes		*1.00*		*1.00*	
No		0.18	0.11-0.28*	0.37	0.19-0.69*
Hormone replacement therapy					
Yes		*1.00*		*1.00*	
No		0.09	0.06-0.14*	0.15	0.08-0.27*
Physician Recommendation					
Diagnostic		*1.00*		*1.00*	
Evaluative		1.23	0.85-1.77	2.00	1.24-3.23*
Breast cancer stage at diagnosis					
Non-advance stage		*1.00*		*1.00*	
Advance stage		0.58	0.41-0.83*	0.69	0.43-1.10
Access to mammogram facilities					
Within 10 miles radius	High access	0.46	0.27-0.77*	0.41	0.22-0.76*
	Medium access	0.42	0.25-0.71*	0.42	0.23-0.76*
	Low access	*1.00*		*1.00*	
Within 20 miles radius	High access	0.60	0.38-0.96*	0.58	0.34-1.00
	Medium access	0.81	0.49-1.35	0.72	0.39-1.31
	Low access	*1.00*		*1.00*	
Within 30 miles radius	High access	0.68	0.42-1.10	0.52	0.29-0.91*
	Medium access	0.67	0.41-1.09	0.85	0.49-1.49
	Low access	*1.00*		*1.00*	

Note. OR = Odds ratio; CI = Confidence interval; * = statistically significant.

(Adjusted Odds ratio for all the independent variables are taken from the logistic model for 30 mile radius)

For the 30 miles radius access measure, women who had high access to mammography facilities was 48% less likely of having had a previous mammogram when compared to women who had less access to mammography facilities (OR = 0.52, 95% CI = 0.29-0.91).

The odds of having had a previous mammogram for women who had high access to mammography facilities were 0.51(95% CI= 0.28-0.92) times compared to women who had less access to mammography facilities and these findings were significant for both the crude and adjusted models developed for the 40 miles radius access measure. The 50 miles radius access measure finding was not statistically significant in any model.

In Table 2, after adjustment for all other variables, women in the age group below 40 years were negatively associated with having had a previous mammogram when compared to women in the age group 40-49 years, which was statistically significant (adjusted OR = 0.11, 95% CI = 0.06-0.22). After adjustment for other variables, neither race nor ethnicity remained significantly associated with having had a previous mammogram when compared with White women. Women's educational attainment level and insurance status were not statistically significantly associated with having had a previous mammogram in the adjusted model. Not having a family history of breast cancer appeared as a negative predictor of having had a previous mammogram in the adjusted model, as it had in the univariate model, and remained statistically significant (adjusted OR = 0.37, 95% CI = 0.19-0.69). The odds of having had a previous mammogram for women who did not have a family history of breast cancer were about one-third as likely as women who had a positive family history of breast cancer. Hormone replacement therapy remained negatively associated with having had a previous mammogram after controlling for all other variables in the adjusted model (adjusted OR = 0.15, 95% CI = 0.08-0.27) and the finding was statistically significant. In the adjusted model after controlling for all other variables, the evaluative recommendation by physicians was found to be a significant predictor of having had a previous mammogram (OR = 2.00, 95% CI = 1.24-3.23).

Discussion

The gravity model, a combined measure of accessibility and availability was used to evaluate the potential spatial interaction between any woman's location and all alternative mammography facilities within a reasonable distance. The relationship of geographical access and utilization of mammogram is noteworthy. In Denver metropolitan area most of mammography facilities are located close to the downtown where accessibility is higher. Women diagnosed with breast cancer without a previous mammogram also higher in this area (Figure 1). In another study we found women diagnosed with advanced stage of breast cancer are also higher in these areas (Rahman, et al., 2007). Several issues contribute in determining which mammography facility to be used to get a mammogram, or more specifically, why a woman would not use the nearest mammography facility or just one facility to obtain her mammograms. Factors such as the type of health insurance and their policies regarding reimbursement may have determined which mammography facility a woman must use to get a mammogram. A common physician practice is to recommend their patients to a specific mammography facility. Some women may prefer to go to a mammography facility that is closer to their work place rather than from their residence. Moreover, it is crucial to specify one mammogram facility that the woman used to measure the straight-line distance from her residence. Typically for a diagnosis of breast cancer a woman will have one or two mammograms and then an ultrasound, which will be followed by a biopsy and all of these examinations usually do not occur within the same clinic or on the same day. Both access and distance are equally important in considering barriers to overcome for screening mammogram and diagnostic testings for breast cancer. Being hindered in either way would likely result in a later stage of breast cancer at diagnosis. Taking into account all the above issues it seems more appropriate that we measure access to mammogram facility considering all the available facilities within an arbitrary radius, rather than the distance from the woman's residence to nearest facility or one specific facility.

Again, in the literature the arbitrary radius is usually considered as 30 miles for FCA method; however most of these studies are about primary care rather than preventive care. Assuming that the minimum distance a woman would be willing to travel to get a preventive service, such as, mammogram would be different, access ratio for several different radii (10, 20, 30, 40, and 50 miles) were measured and compared. While comparing access measures of different arbitrary radiuses in the FCA method, as the radius increased from 10 miles to 50 miles, the standard deviation of access measures decreased and also the range from minimum to maximum decreased (Table 3).

This indicates that the access measure with a higher radius had less variance, which led to stronger spatial smoothing, which is a manifestation of MAUP (modifiable areal unit problem). Access scores tended to increase with increasing radius, as one would have more access if she were permitted or capable of traveling further. As the radius increased from 10 miles to 50 miles, the population with high access also increased (Figure 2, Figure 3 and Figure 4).

Table 3. Comparison of Accessibility Measures

Radius	Total number	Minimum	Maximum	Mean	Std. Deviation
10 Mile	1745	.0000000	.1075926	.0263610	.0261128
20 Mile	1745	.0000000	.0768412	.0263610	.0136416
30 Mile	1745	.0000000	.0536146	.0263610	.0084047
40 Mile	1745	.0000000	.0377056	.0263610	.0056572
50 Mile	1745	.0011524	.0314764	.0263610	.0042359

N= 2042.
Frequency missing 297.

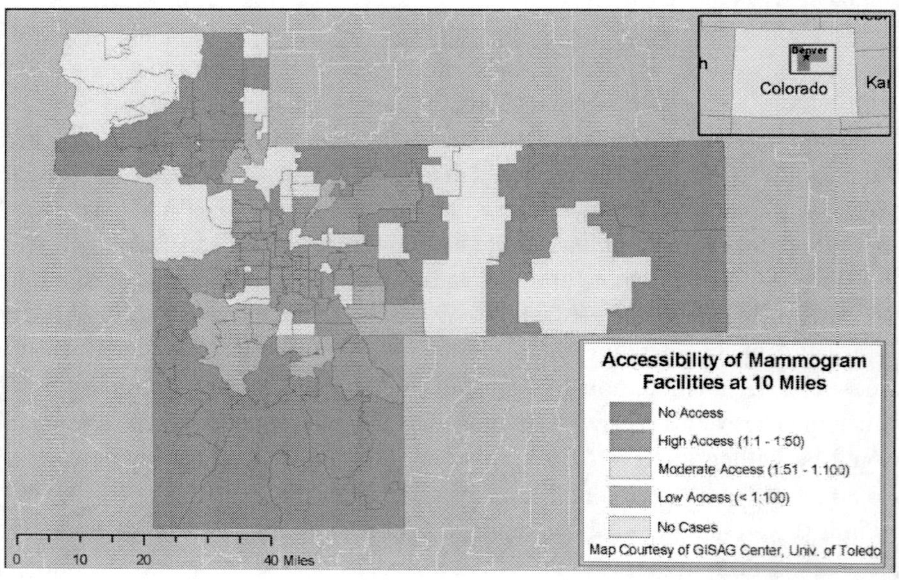

Figure 2. Accessibility to Mammogram Facilities within 10 Miles Radius (by Zip Code).

However, if we look at the mean access measure for the population, it remains the same for all the measures with different radiuses (Table 3) as because increasing radius does not necessarily mean increasing access. Access depends on the distribution of supply of and demand for mammograms. In the method of calculating access to mammography facilities in the current study, the availability of the facility was considered only by the total number of women sharing that facility, which meant that all the mammography facilities were viewed as having equal capacity. When the radius increased, the number of women within that arbitrary radius increased as well, which acted to decrease the ultimate access to a mammography facility as more women shared that facility. To overcome this limitation, future research is needed that will consider the qualitative aspects of the mammography facilities, such as, the size, number of staff members, amount of equipment and other details that might have affected the capacity of a facility.

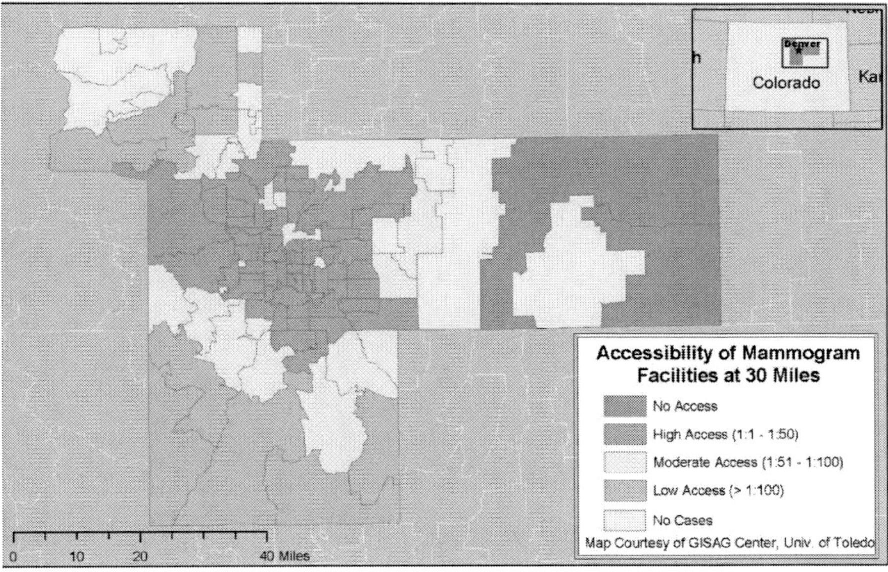

Figure 3. Accessibility to Mammogram Facilities within 30 Miles Radius (by Zip Code).

Several other limitations that were related to the access measure of the current study are as follows: First, the population data were geocoded by using women's Zip codes as exact addresses were not available because of a requirement to maintain confidentiality. By using Zip codes, women were assigned to an area rather than assigned to a single point. This technique might have decreased the level of precision for the measure of access to mammography facility. Second, the current study was limited to only six county areas. A known limitation of the FCA method in measuring access is that people within a catchment area have equal access to all providers within that same catchment area, and all providers beyond the radius of the catchment area are inaccessible, regardless of any differences in distances (Luo, 2004; Luo and Wang, 2004;). Finally, absence of individual level data on income or socio-economic status and missing data on health insurance, education, hormone replacement therapy, family history, physician recommendation and previous mammogram were also a major limitation of the current study.

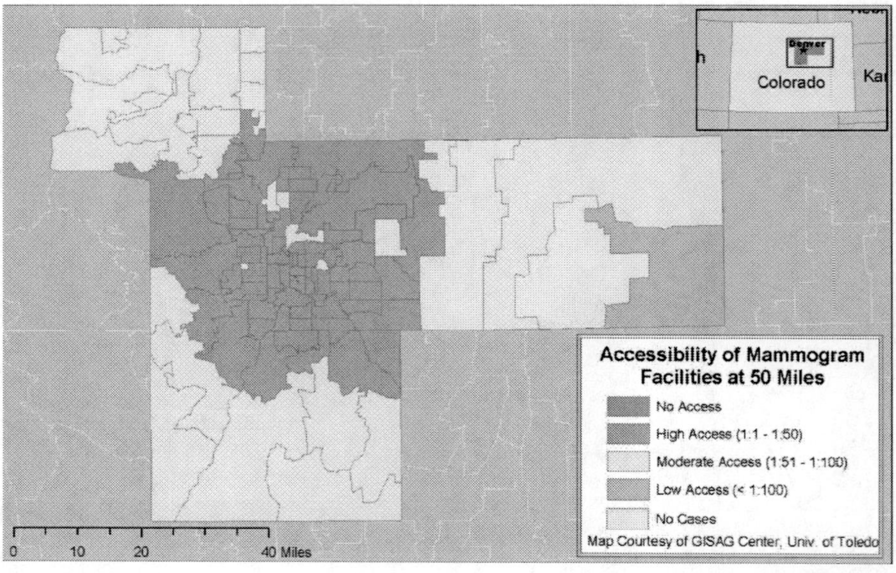

Figure 4. Accessibility to Mammogram Facilities within 50 Miles Radius (by Zip Code).

ACKNOWLEDGEMENT

Dr. Fahui Wang, Department of Geography, Northern Illinois University.

REFERENCES

American Cancer Society: *Cancer Facts and Figure ures 2003-2004*. Atlanta, American Cancer Society, Inc, 2005.

Ann, B.N., Ronald, T.K., Raymond, G.H., and Gilligan, M.A. (2001). Relationship of distance from a radiotherapy facility and initial breast cancer treatment. *Journal of National Cancer Institute. 93(17),* 1344-1346.

Blanchard, K., Colbert, J.A., Puri, D., Weissman, J., Moy, B., Kopans, D.B. et al. (2004). Mammographic screening: Patterns of use and estimated impact on breast carcinoma survival. *Cancer, 101,* 495-507.

Croner, C.M., Sperling, J., and Broome, F. R. (1996). Geographic information systems (GIS): New perspectives in understanding human health and environmental relationships. *Statistics in Medicine, 15,* 1961-1977.

Duffy, S., Taber, L., Chen, H.H., Smith, A., Holmberg, L., Jonsson, H., et al., (2006). Reduction in Breast Cancer Mortality from Organized Service Screening with Mammography: 1. Further Confirmation with Extended Data. *Cancer Epidemiol Biomarkers Prev, 15(1),* 45–51.

Duffy, S., Taber, L., and Chen, H.H. (2002). The impact of organized mammographic service screening on breast cancer mortality in seven Swedish counties. *Cancer, 95,* 458-469.

Edwards, B.K., Howe, H.L., Ries, L.A.G., Thun, M.J., Rosenberg, H.M., Yancik, R., et al. (2002). Annual report to the Nation on the status of cancer, 1973-1999, featuring implications of age and aging on US cancer burden. *Cancer, 94,* 2766-2792.

Fortney, J., Rost, K., and Warren, J. (2003). Comparing alternative methods of measuring geographic access to health services. *Health Services and Outcomes Research Methodology.* 1(2): 173-184.

Goodman, D., Fisher, E., Stukel, T., and Chang, C. (1997). The distance to community medical care and the likelihood of hospitalization: Is closer always better? *Am. J. Public Health, 87,*144–50.

Haynes, R., Bentham, G., Lovett, A., and Gale, S. (1999). Effects of distances to hospital and GP surgery on hospital inpatient episodes controlling for needs and provision. *Soc. Sci. Med, 49,* 425–433.

Howe, H. L., Wingo, P. A., Thun, M. J., Ries, L. A. G., Rosenberg, H. M., Feigal, E.G. et al. (2001). Annual report to the nation on the status of cancer (1973 through 1998), features cancers with recent increasing trends. *J. Natl. Cancer Inst, 93,* 824-842.

Humphrey, L.L., Helfand, M., Chan, B.K., Woolf, S.H. (2002). Breast cancer screening: a summary of the evidence for the U.S. Preventive Services Task Force. *Ann. Intern. Med., 137(5),* 347-360.

Jilda, C.G., Hyndman, C. D'Arcy, and Holman, J. (2000a). Differential effects on socioeconomic groups of modelling the location of mammography screening clinics using geographic information systems. *Australian and New Zealand Journal of Public Health, 24(3),* 281-286.

Jilda, C.G., Hyndman, C. D'Arcy, and Holman, J. (2000b). Effect of distance and social disadvantage on the response to invitations to attend mammography screening. *J. Med. Screen, 7,* 141-145.

Joseph, A., and Phillips, D. (1984). *Accessibility and Utilization: Geographical Perspectives on Health Care Delivery.* New York: Harper and Row.

Khan, A. A. and Bhardwaj, S. M. (1994). Access to health care: A conceptual framework and its relevance to health care planning. *Evaluation and the Health Professions. 17(1)* : 60-76.

Luo, W. (2004). Using a GIS-based floating catchment method to assess areas with shortage of physicians. *Health and Place, 10,* 1-11.

Luo, W., and Wang, F. (2003). Measures of spatial accessibility to health care in a GIS environment: synthesis and a case study in the Chicago region. *Environment and Planning B: Planning and Design, 30,* 865-884.

Rahman, S., Price, J. M., Dignan, M., Rahman, S. M., Lindquist, P. S., and Jordan, T. M. (2007). Access to mammography facilities and breast cancer stage at diagnosis: A GIS approach. Paper accepted for oral presentation at the AACE Annual Meeting 2007 (Oct 11-13): Cancer Education in Minority and Underserved Populations. UAB Comprehensive Cancer Center, Alabama.

Smith, R.A., Saslow, D., Sawyer, K.A., Burke, W., Costanza, M.E., Evans, W.P., et al.(2003). American Cancer Society guidelines for breast cancer screening: Update 2003. *CA Cancer J. Clin., 53(3),* 141-169.

Tabar, L., Yen, M.F., Vitak, B., Chen, H.H., Smith, R.A., and Duffy, S.W. (2003). Mammography service screening and mortality in breast cancer patients: 20-year follow-up before and after introduction of screening. *Lancet, 361(9367),* 1405-1410.

Williams, W.H., Holladay, D.A., and Sheikh, A.A., et al. (2003). Practical impact of screening mammography: Analysis of Pathological factors and treatment utilization for women undergoing breast conservation therapy at a large radiation therapy center. *Proc. Am. Soc. Clin. Oncol. , 22,* 87-95.

INDEX

A

B

C

D

E

F

G

N

O

P

Q

R

S

T

U

V

W

X

Y